DIAGNOSTIC PICTURE TESTS IN

Hematology

DIAGNOSTIC PICTURE TESTS IN

Hematology

Alastair J. Bellingham
FRCP, PRCPath
Professor of Haematology
King's College Hospital
London, UK

Henry Hambley
Bsc(Hons), MBChB, MRCPath
Consultant Haematologist
King's College Hospital
London, UK

M Mosby-Wolfe

London Baltimore Bogotá Boston Buenos Aires Caracas Carlsbad, CA Chicago Madrid Mexico City Milan Naples, FL
New York Philadelphia St. Louis Sydney Tokyo Toronto Wiesbaden

02682252

Project Manager:	Alison Taylor
Development Editor:	Jennifer Prast
Production:	Jane Tozer
Index:	Jill Halliday
Publisher:	Richard Furn

Copyright © 1995 Times Mirror International Publishers Limited.

Published in 1995 by Mosby-Wolfe, an imprint of Times Mirror International Publishers Limited.

Printed in Italy by Imago Publishing Ltd.

ISBN 0 7234 1936 1

09 MAP 1998

To Jill

Preface

We live in a time of change. Both undergraduate and post-graduate medical education are planned for radical restructure in the next few years. During a time of change it is imperative that current trainees are not undersold. In producing this book, which is primarily aimed at undergraduates and those entering basic specialist training, we have endeavoured to demonstrate both the scientific basis and the inextricably linked clinical and laboratory aspects of haematology.

It is the latter which is so attractive to enthusiasts, and we hope that others will find it likewise.

Alastair Bellingham
Henry Hambley

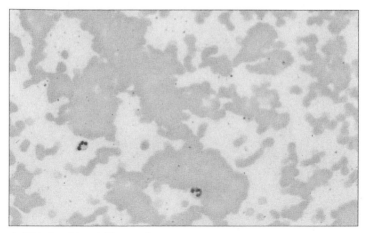

1. This is a blood film made at room temperature. What does it show and what is the significance?

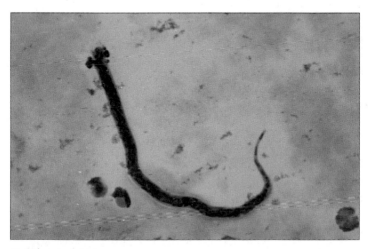

2. What is this?

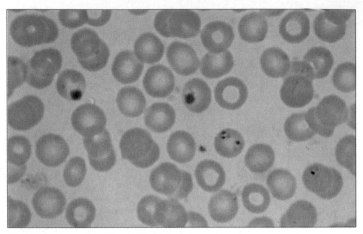

3. What does this blood film show?

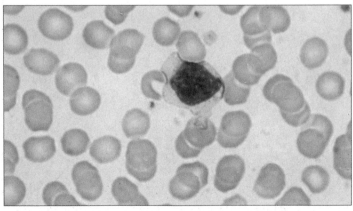

4. The blood film from a 14-year-old boy complaining of fever and sore throat. What does this show and what diagnostic test should be done?

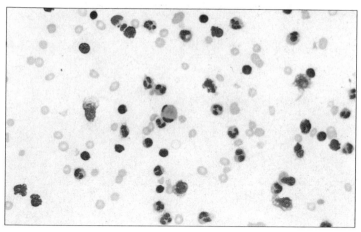

5. What is this?

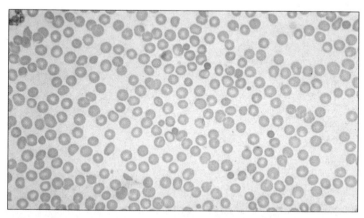

6. This blood film is from a 25-year-old man who has noticed occasional episodes of jaundice over many years, often associated with intercurrent infections. What abnormality is seen on the blood film and what is the likely diagnosis?

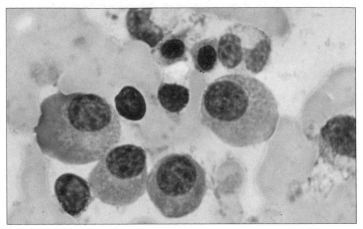

7. This is a marrow smear from a 72-year-old man with a pathological fracture of his humerus. What is the diagnosis?

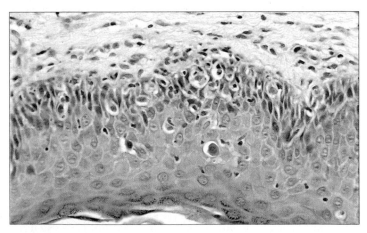

8. This is a skin biopsy from a patient 30 days post-allogenic bone marrow transplant. What is the diagnosis?

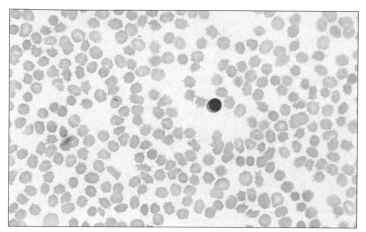

9. What are these red cells?

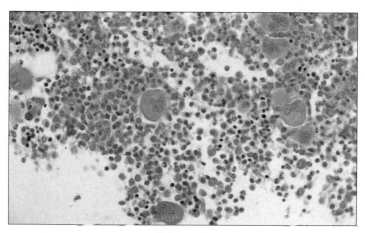

10. This is a marrow biopsy from a patient with a platelet count of 1000 x 10⁹/l. What is the diagnosis?

11. What is shown?

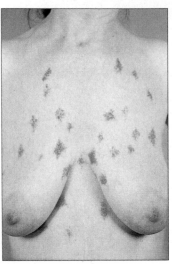

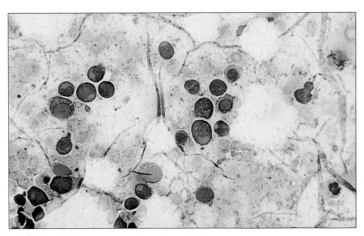

12. Marrow shows increased numbers of blasts and has been stained with sudan black B. What is shown?

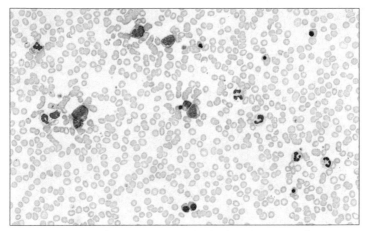

13. What are the film appearances and what may cause these?

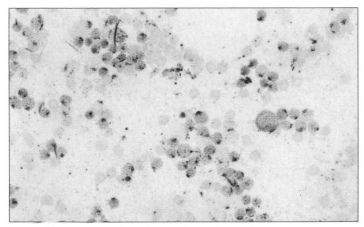

14. Marrow with increased numbers of blasts stained with acid phosphatase. What is the significance of this appearance?

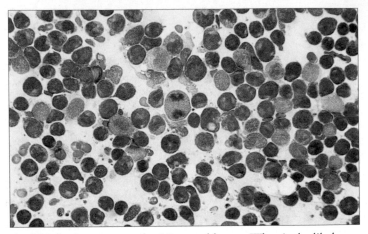

15. This is the marrow of a 64-year-old man. What is the likely diagnosis?

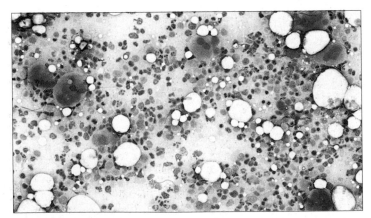

16. This is a marrow from a 35-year-old woman who presented with widespread purpura and a platelet count of 5 x 10⁹/l. What is the likely diagnosis?

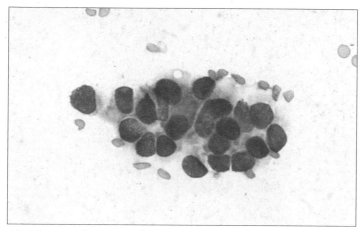

17. Marrow of a man with a leucoerythroblastic blood film. What is the diagnosis?

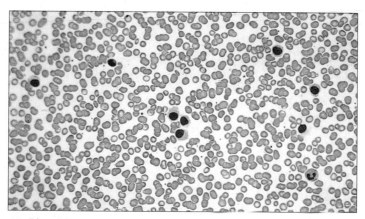

18. Blood film from a man who presented with pancytopenia. He was found to have marked splenomegaly. What is the likely diagnosis?

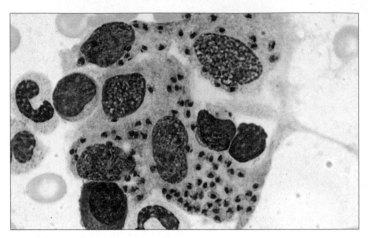

19. What is this?

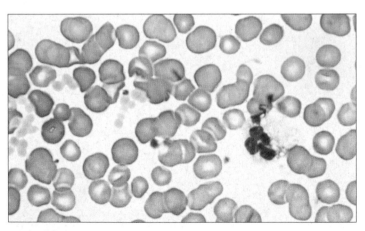

20. This is a blood film from a man whose white cell count was reported as 25 x 10^9/l by an automated counter. What is the diagnosis?

21. CT scan of a chest. What is the diagnosis?

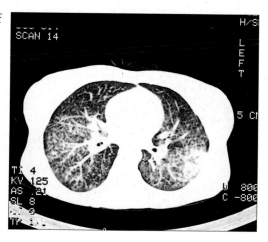

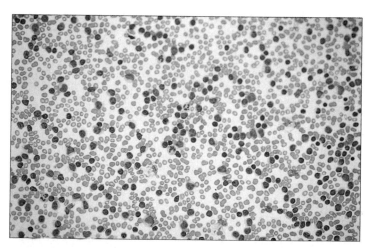

22. This is a blood film from a 75-year-old man admitted for prostatectomy. What is the diagnosis?

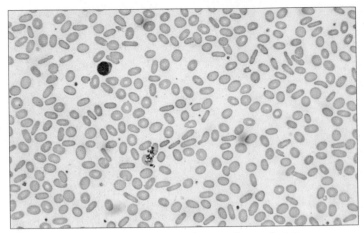

23. Is this condition associated with severe haemolysis?

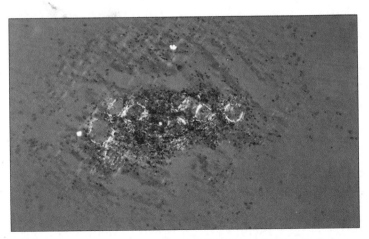

24. Bone marrow aspirate stained with sirius red. What is the diagnosis?

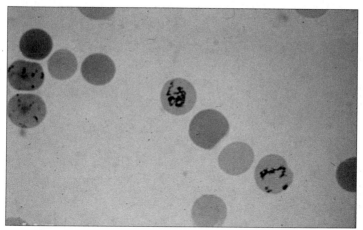

25. What cells are shown here?

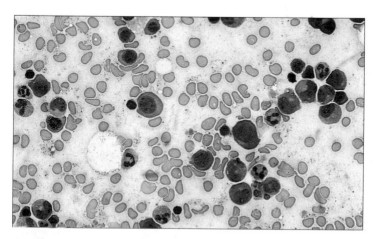

26. This is a marrow from a 67-year-old woman. What is the diagnosis?

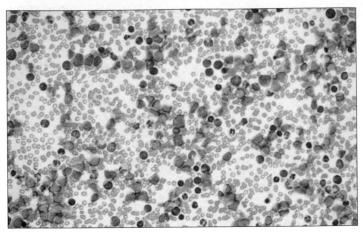

27. This is a blood film from a 34-year-old woman who has had chronic leukaemia for the past three years. What has happened?

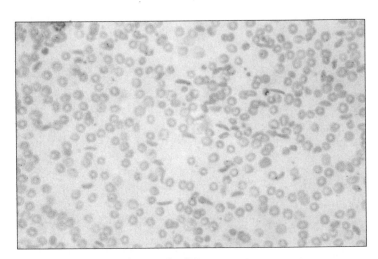

28. What are these abnormal cells?

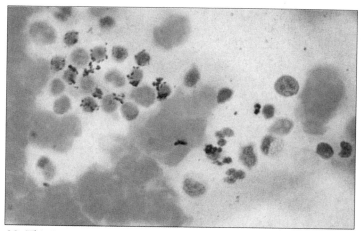

29. This is an iron-stained marrow from a 45-year-old man with a six month history of increasing tiredness and breathlessness. What is the diagnosis?

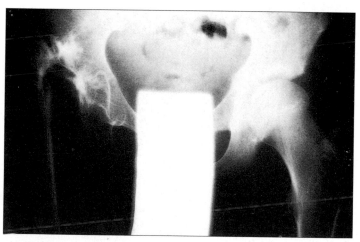

30. What does this show?

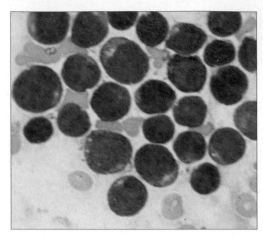

31. This is a marrow aspirate from a 16-year-old male who was noted to have lymphadenopathy. What is the diagnosis?

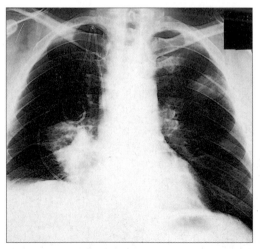

32. This is a chest x-ray from a 48-year-old man undergoing intensive chemotherapy for non-Hodgkin's lymphoma. He had been neutropenic and afebrile for two weeks and had received several different combinations of broad spectrum antibiotics. What does the x-ray show and what is the likely diagnosis?

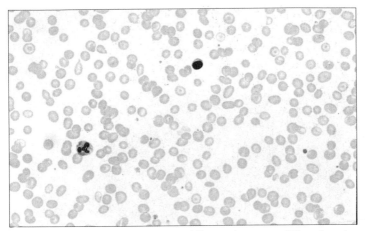

33. This is a blood film from a middle-aged woman. What does it show?

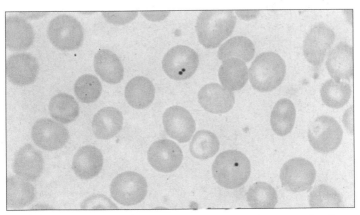

34. Blood film from a 34-year-old man admitted to Casualty. An abdominal scar was noted on examination. What abnormalities are seen?

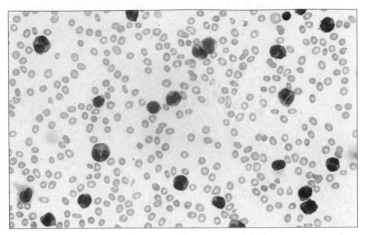

35. Blood film from a 68-year-old man noted to be anaemic and bruised. What is the diagnosis?

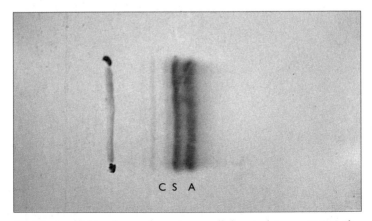

C S A

36. Haemoglobin electrophoresis on cellular acetate at pH 8.6; the black dots mark the origin. The position of haemoglobins A, S and C is shown below. What does this show ?

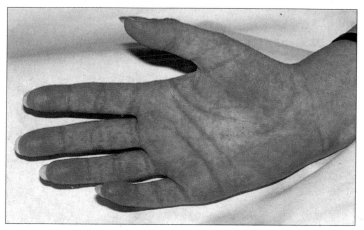

37. This is a hand of a patient who is 30 days post-allogeneic bone marrow transplant. What does it show and what is the diagnosis?

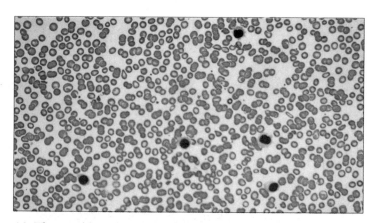

38. This is a blood film from a 58-year-old woman who was noted to be anaemic, thrombocytopenic and leucopenic. Splenomegaly was noted on examination, although there was no lymphadenopathy. A marrow aspirate failed to yield any particles. What does the blood film show and what is the likely diagnosis?

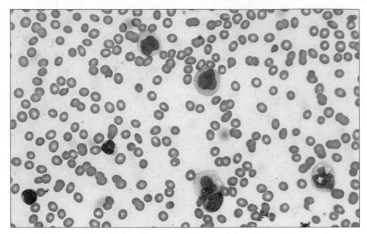

39. This is a blood film from a 46-year-old woman who complained of bleeding gums and attended her dentist. The dentist noticed gum hypertrophy and referred her for a full blood count. What is the likely diagnosis?

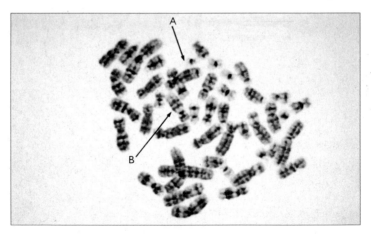

40. This is a chromosome preparation from a 42-year-old patient with splenomegaly. What is shown?

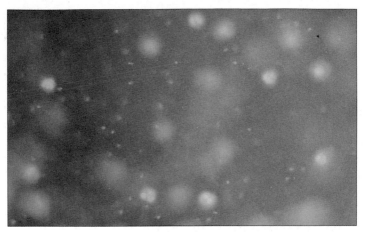

41. This is a film of buffy court stained with acridine orange and photographed under fluorescence. What does it show?

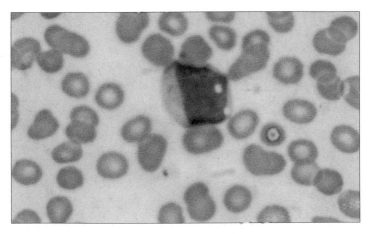

42. This is a blood film from a patient with acute leukaemia. What does it show?

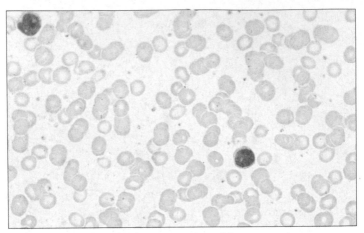

43. This is a blood film from a 36-year-old woman who was found to be slightly anaemic during pregnancy. What does it show and what is the diagnosis?

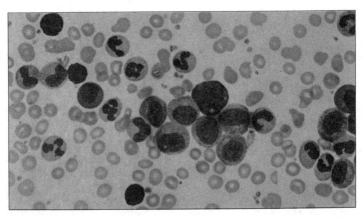

44. This is a blood film from a patient with a white cell count of 84 x 10⁹/l. On examination the patient was noted to have moderate splenomegaly. What is the diagnosis?

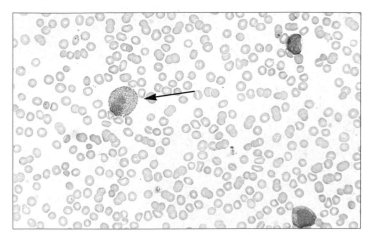

45. What is this cell?

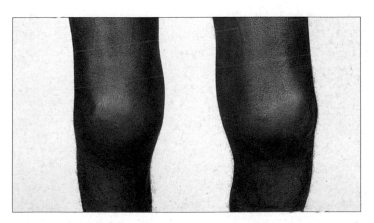

46. The knees of a 27-year-old African who complained of recurrent joint pain are shown. What does the slide show and what is the likely diagnosis?

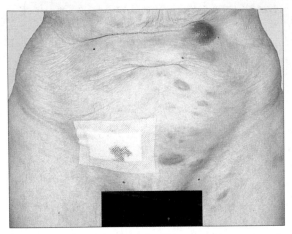

47. This is the abdomen of a 79-year-old woman who was known to have polycythaemia rubra vera for 15 years. Recently she became anaemic and had noticed the sudden appearance of lumps on the skin. What are these and what does this change imply?

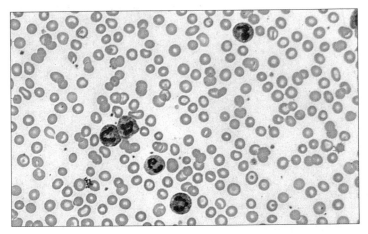

48. This is a blood film from a patient with lobar pneumonia. What does it show?

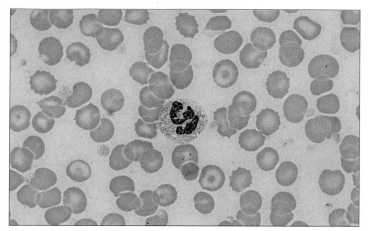

49. This is a blood film from a patient with a mean corpuscular volume (MCV) of 120 fl. What is the likely cause of this?

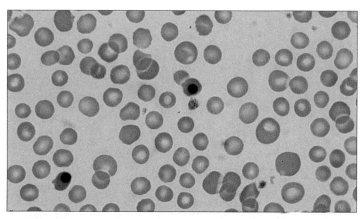

50. This is a blood film from a neonate who was noted to be jaundiced shortly after birth. What does this blood film show and what is the likely diagnosis?

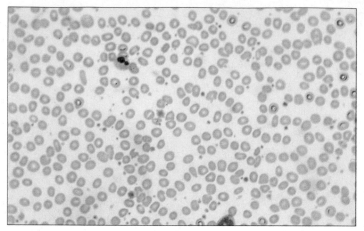

51. This is a blood film from a patient who presented with a stroke. What does it show?

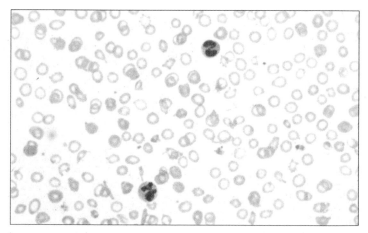

52. This is a blood film from a patient who failed a copper sulphate test at a blood donating session. What does it show?

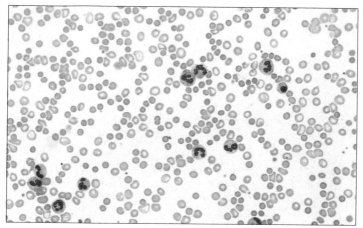

53. This is a blood film from a seven-year-old child who was noted to be pale and slightly jaundiced. What is the diagnosis?

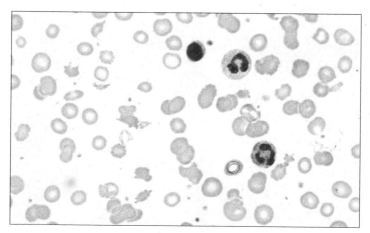

54. This is a blood film from a 34-year-old woman who is in acute renal failure. What is shown?

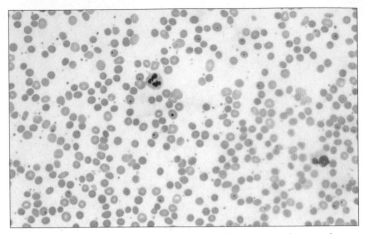

55. This is a blood film from a 55-year-old woman who is pale and jaundiced. What is the diagnosis?

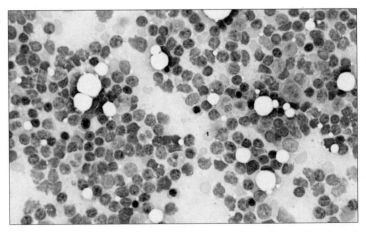

56. This is a marrow film from a patient with a white cell count of 100 x 10⁹/l. What does it show and what is the likely diagnosis?

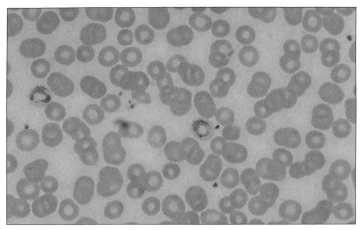

57. This is a blood film from a patient who was found to be afebrile having returned from the Middle East. What does it show?

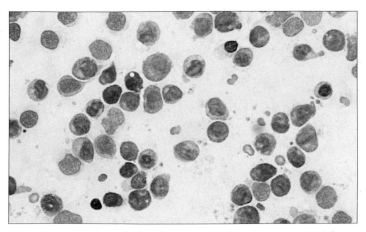

58. This is a marrow from a 63-year-old man who presented with pancytopenia. What does it show and what is the likely diagnosis?

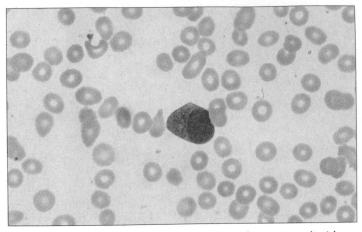

59. This is a blood film from a young man who presented with anaemia, bleeding from gums and marked purpura. What does it show?

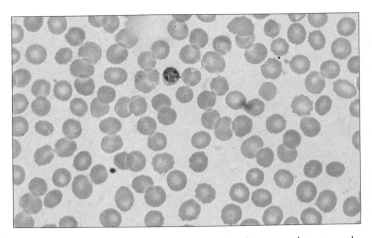

60. This is a blood film from a patient who has recently returned from West Africa. What is the diagnosis?

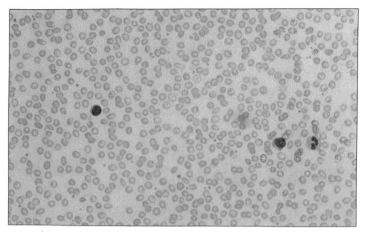

61. This is a blood film from a 22-year-old woman who is pregnant. She was found to be mildly anaemic with a haemoglobin of 12g/dl and mean corpuscular volume (MCV) of 64fl. What is the diagnosis?

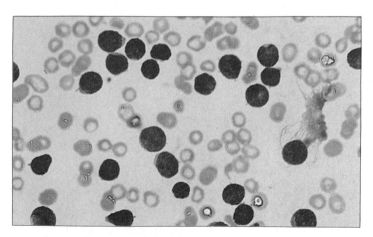

62. This is a blood film from a seven-year-old boy who presents with anaemia and neutropenia. What is the likely diagnosis?

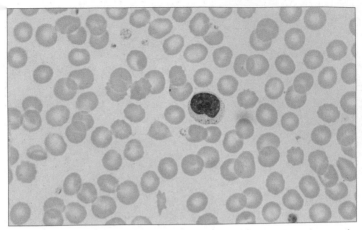

63. This is a blood film from a patient who has splenomegaly and is noted to be neutropenic. What is the diagnosis?

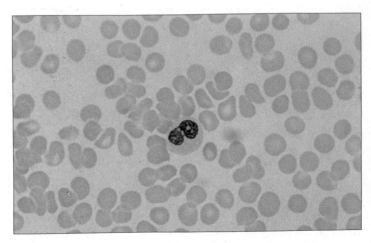

64. What is this cell?

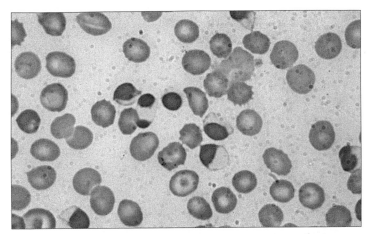

65. This is a blood film from a 7-year-old Italian boy who has had several episodes of jaundice. What does the film show and what is the likely diagnosis. How would this be confirmed?

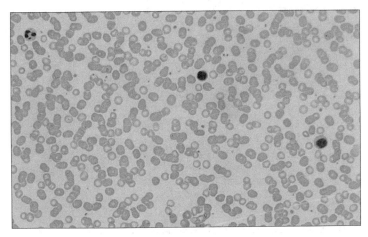

66. What does this blood film show?

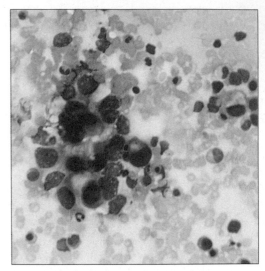

67. These are two views of a marrow aspirate at high power. The top one is stained with an MGG stain and the lower one with a PAS technique. What is the diagnosis?

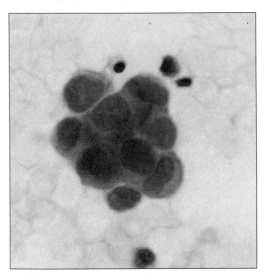

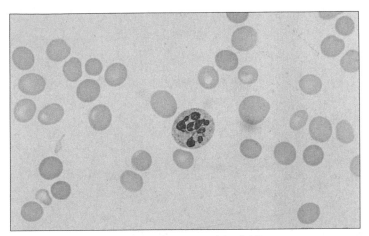

68. What is the cell shown in the centre of the field?

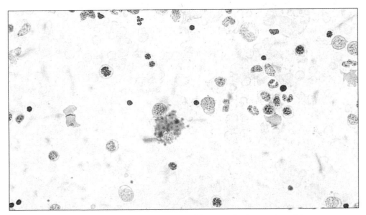

69. This is a marrow smear stained by Perl's Prussian blue reaction for iron. What is shown and what further investigations should be done?

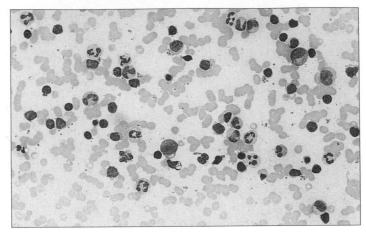

70. This is a marrow aspirate film from a 75-year-old woman who was found to have an IgM paraprotein. What does this show and what is the likely diagnosis?

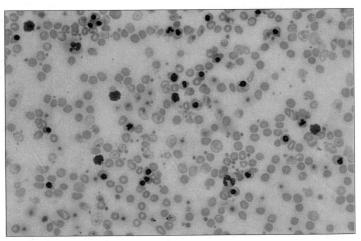

71. This is a blood film from a four-year-old girl from Cyprus who was noted to have massive splenomegaly. What does the blood film show and what is the diagnosis?

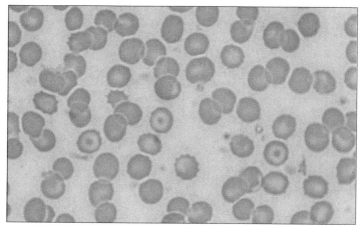

72. What are these red cells and what is the cause of this change?

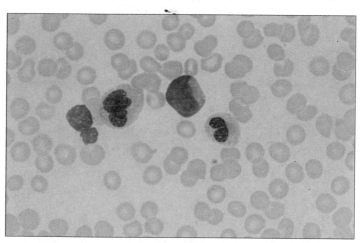

73. This is a blood film from a 72-year-old man who was diagnosed as having polycythaemia rubra vera 15 years ago. He had been treated with venesection and radioactive phosphorus. He had been well until 3 months ago when it was noted that his haemoglobin and platelet counts were falling and his white cell count was rising. What does the blood film show and what does this represent?

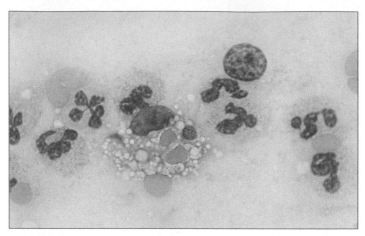

74. This is a marrow from a patient with an opacity on the chest x-ray. What does it show and what would be the likely diagnosis?

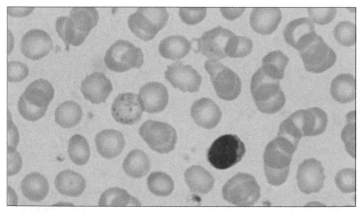

75. Blood film from a 46-year-old male demolition worker admitted with abdominal pain. What does it show and what is the diagnosis?

76. What has happened here? What treatment is required?

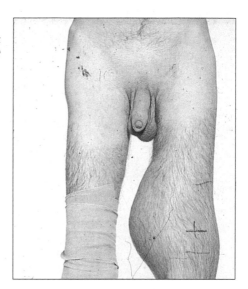

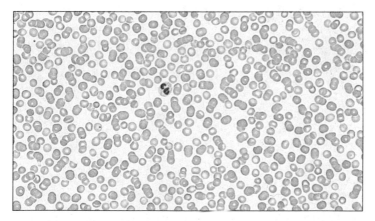

77. This is a blood film from a 7-year-old boy with a purpuric rash affecting his lower legs. What is shown and what is the likely diagnosis?

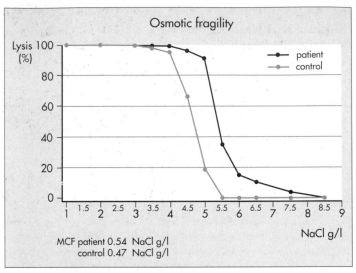

78. This is an osmotic fragility curve. What does it show?

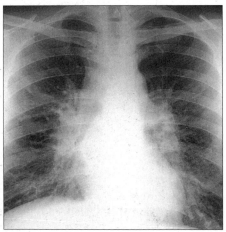

79. This is an x-ray from a 23-year-old woman who has noticed some cervical lymphadenopathy for three months. What abnormalities are seen and what diagnoses may be likely?

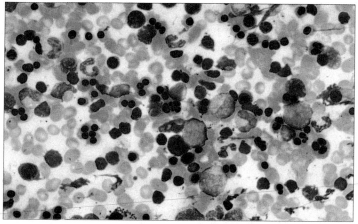

80. This is a bone marrow from a one-year-old child who was found to be anaemic. What does it show and what further investigations could be done to confirm the diagnosis?

81. Picture of the head and neck of a man who complains of dyspnoea. What is shown and what is the likely diagnosis?

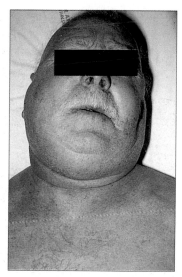

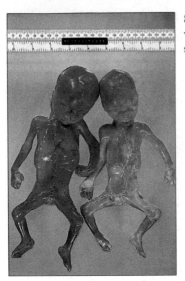

82. This is a picture of twins who died *in utero*. What is shown?

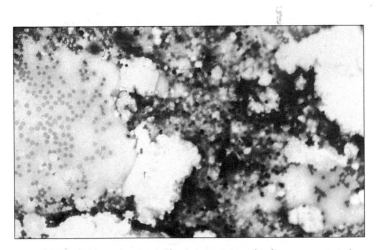

83. This is the bone marrow from a patient who became pancytopenic. What is shown?

84. What is the diagnosis?

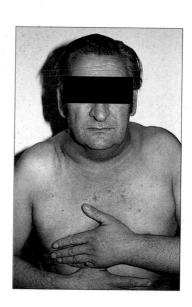

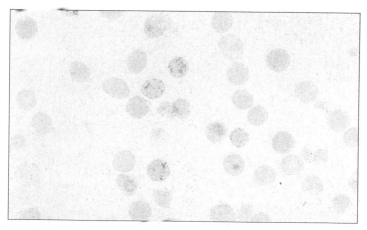

85. This is a blood film stained with crystal violet. What does it show?

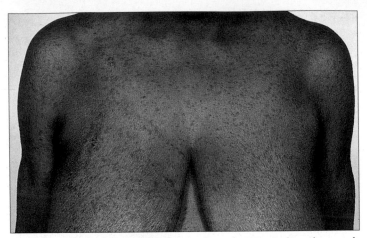

86. This is the upper chest of a woman from the West Indies who noted a rash appearing over the last six weeks. Examination also revealed lymphadenopathy and the blood film showed atypical lymphocytes. The serum Ca^{++} was raised. What is the likely diagnosis?

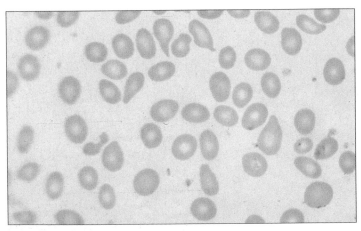

87. This is a blood film from a patient with marked splenomegaly. What is the diagnosis?

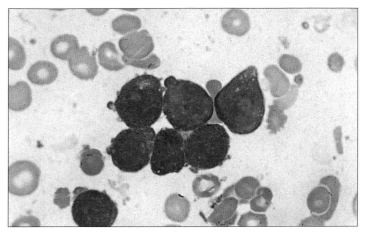

88. This is a marrow from an elderly man who was found to be anaemic with a haemoglobin of 5g/dl. What does it show and what diagnosis is likely?

89. This is a middle-aged man. What is the likely diagnosis?

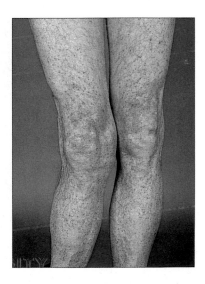

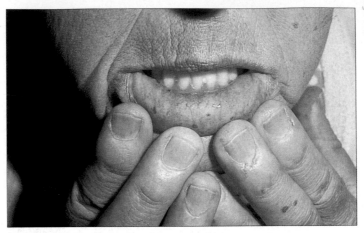

90. What is shown here and how would it present?

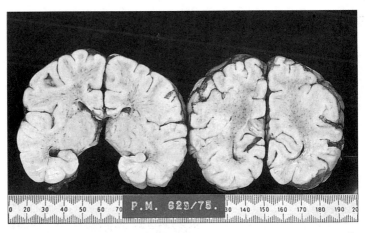

P.M. 629/75.

91. This is a cut surface of the brain taken from a post mortem of a child who died at one month of age. What is shown?

92. This is a lumbar spine x-ray from a young man complaining of back pain. What is shown and what could be causing this?

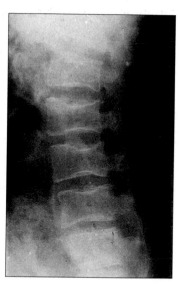

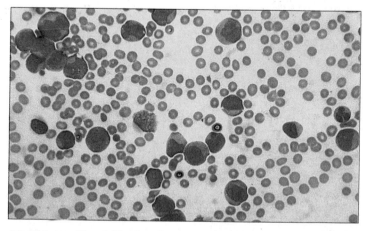

93. This is a blood film from a patient aged 46 years who was found to be anaemic. What is the diagnosis?

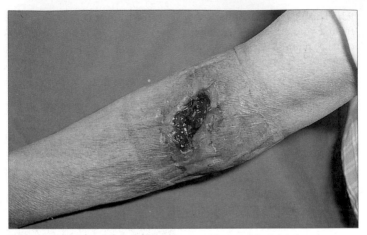

94. This is the forearm of a patient with non-Hodgkin's lymphoma. What has happened?

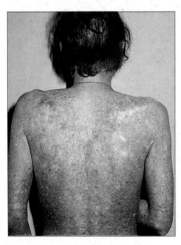

95. This patient had an allogeneic bone marrow transplantation four months ago. What is shown and what is the diagnosis?

96. These pictures show the face and hands of a woman with lymphadenopathy. What is shown and what is the diagnosis?

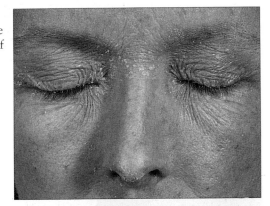

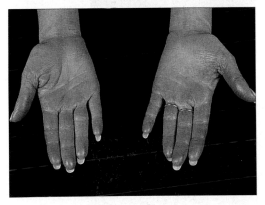

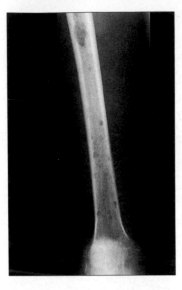

97. This is an x-ray of a femur of a 67-year-old man who complains of pain in the lower leg. What is shown and what is the likely diagnosis?

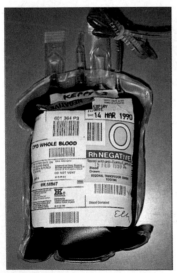

98. What is this and what would it be used for?

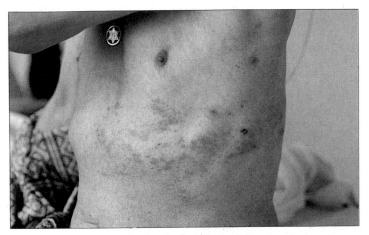

99. What is shown and what is the diagnosis?

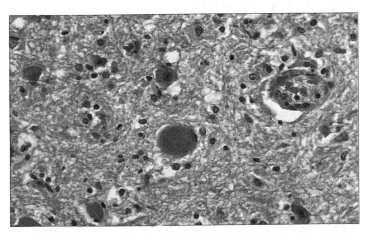

100. This is a section of lymph node from a patient with generalised lymphadenopathy. What is shown?

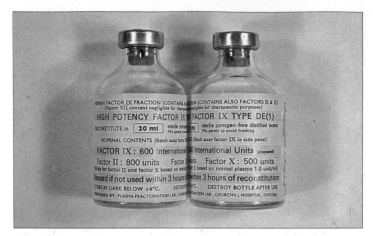

101. What is this?

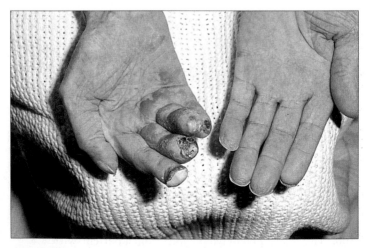

102. What is shown here? What could be the diagnosis?

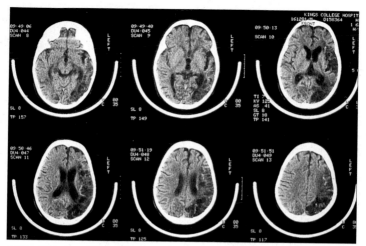

103. This is a CT head scan of a five-year-old girl who has sickle cell disease. What is shown?

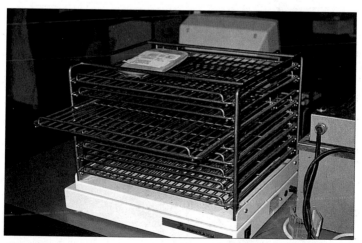

104. What is this and what would it be used for?

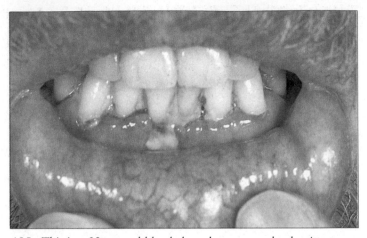

105. This is a 32-year-old bachelor who went to the dentist because of bleeding gums. A subsequent full blood count was normal. What is the diagnosis?

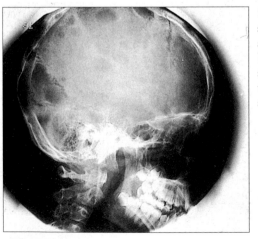

106. This is a skull x-ray from a 16-year-old boy. What does it show and what is the likely diagnosis?

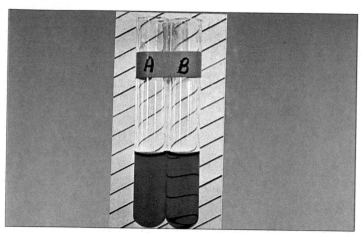

107. What is this?

108. This is a chest x-ray from a young man with sickle cell disease who complains of chest pain and breathlessness. What is the differential diagnosis?

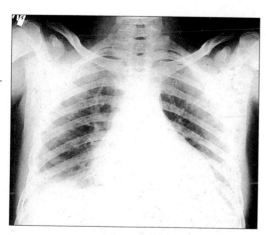

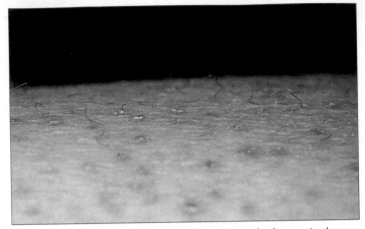

109. This is a picture of a forearm of a patient who has noticed some easy bruising. What does it show and what is the likely diagnosis?

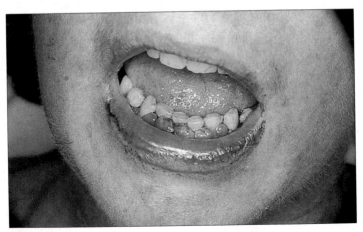

110. This young woman complained of bleeding gums. What is the likely diagnosis?

111. This is an arteriogram and the resected kidney of a patient who was found to be polycythaemic. What is shown and what is the cause?

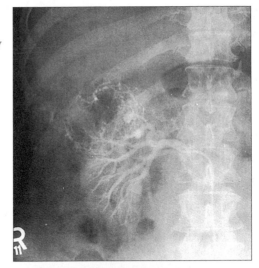

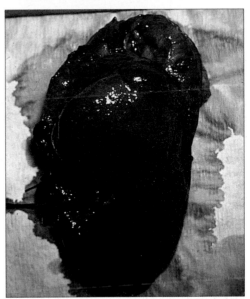

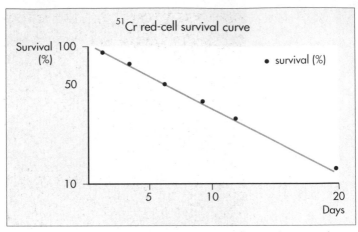

112. This shows a red-cell survival curve. What is shown and what would be a likely explanation for this?

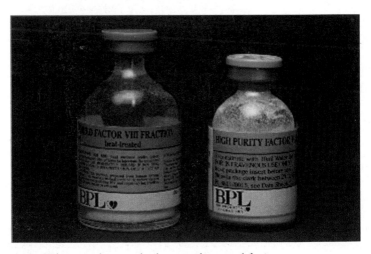

113. What are these and what are they used for?

114. What is this?

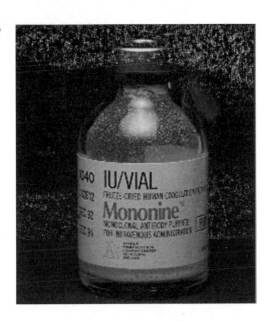

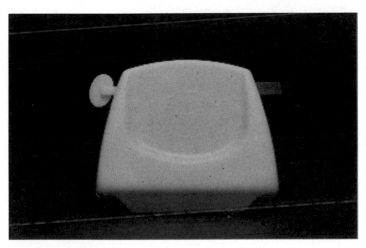

115. What is this device and what is it used for?

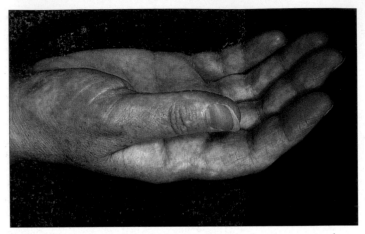

116. What is shown here in this woman who has just received chemotherapy for acute myeloid leukaemia?

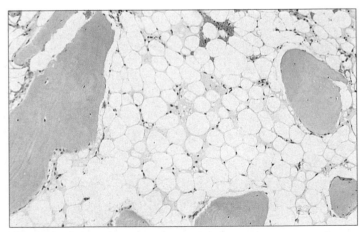

117. This is a bone marrow trephine from a patient who is pancytopenic. What does it show?

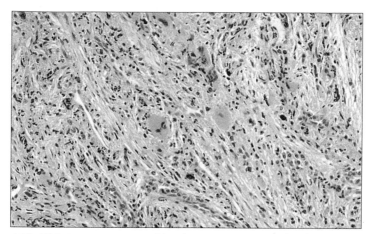

118. This is a marrow trephine from a patient noted to have splenomegaly. What does it show?

119. This is a picture of the retina. What is shown?

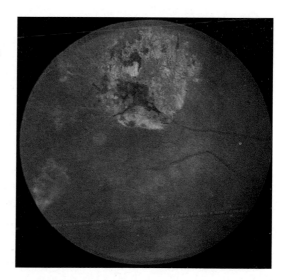

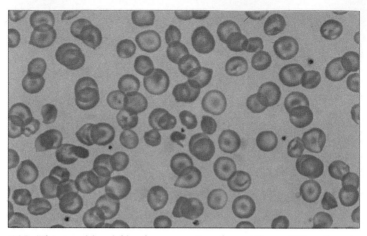

120. This is a blood film from a patient from Ghana. What does it show?

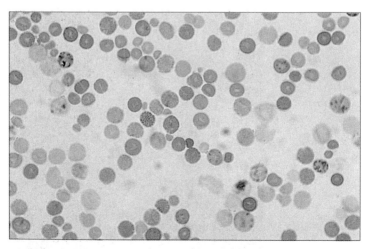

121. Blood film stained with cresyl blue. What does it show?

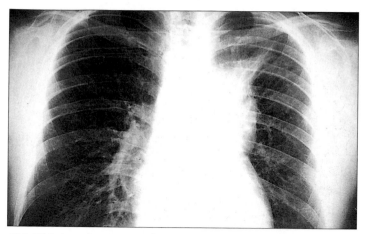

122. This is a chest x-ray of a patient who complained of breathlessness. What is the likely cause of this appearance?

123. What does this skull x-ray show?

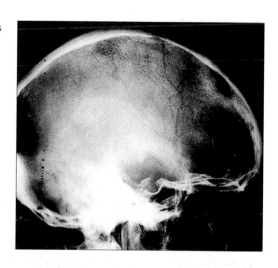

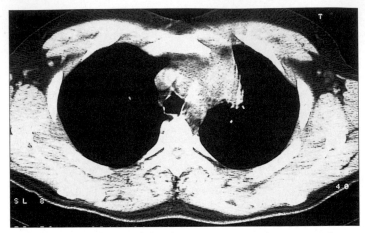

124. This is a CT scan of the chest in a patient who presented with cervical lymphadenopathy. What is shown?

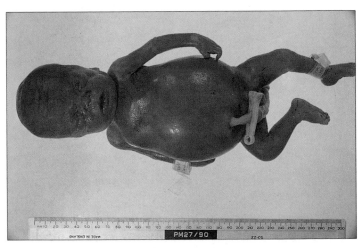

125. What is this and what could be a likely cause?

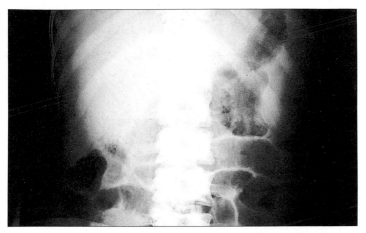

126. This is an abdominal x-ray taken from a patient who often complained of right-sided abdominal pain. What does it show and how does it explain the abdominal pain? What is the underlying diagnosis?

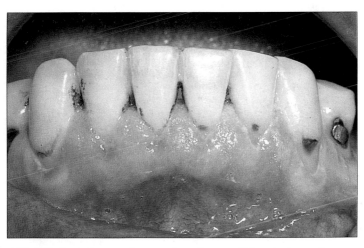

127. This is a picture of a mouth and gums. What is shown?

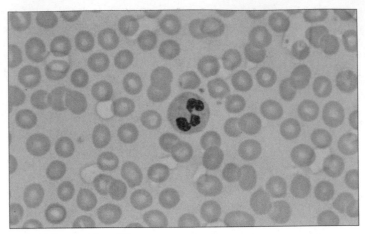

128. What is this cell?

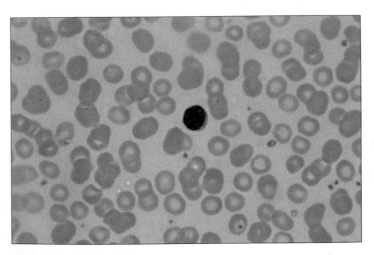

129. What is this cell?

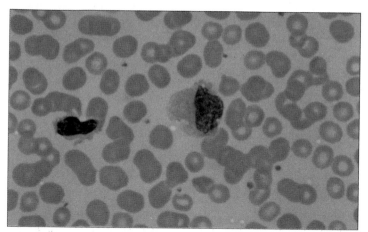

130. What is this cell?

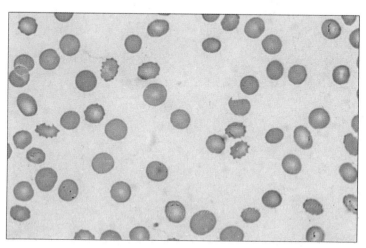

131. What is this cell?

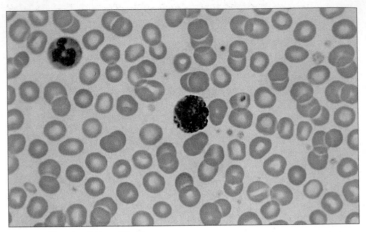

132. What is this cell?

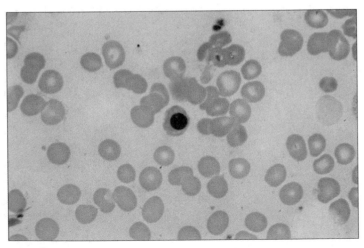

133. What is this cell?

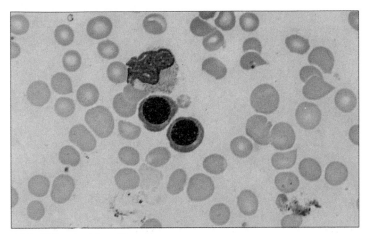

134. What is this cell?

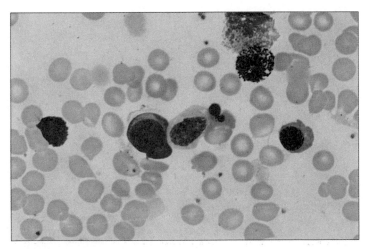

135. What is this cell?

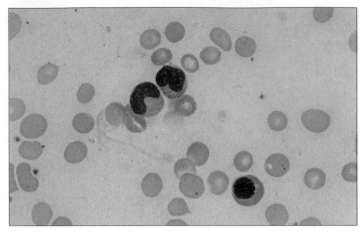

136. What is this cell?

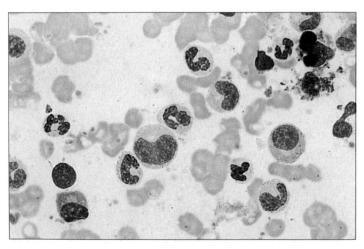

137. What is this cell?

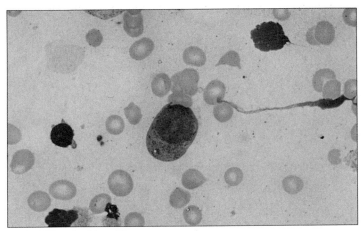

138. What is this cell?

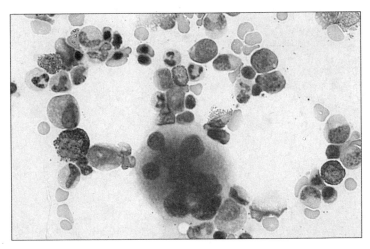

139. What is this cell?

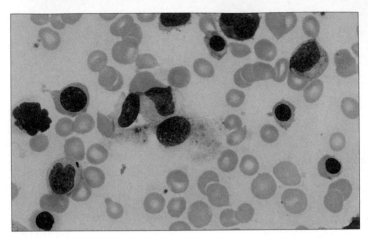

140. What is this cell?

Answers

1. This blood film shows agglutination of red cells due to the presence of cold haemagglutonin. This may be a primary phenomenon or secondary to infection or lymphoma.

2. This is a parasite, Loa Loa. This is one of a number of microfilaria which cause swelling of tissues, classically elephantiasis, and lymphadenopathy. The microfilaria may be difficult to find since they are often found in peripheral blood only at certain times of the day. They have characteristic morphology but it is advisable to have the species confirmed at a centre specialising in tropical diseases.

3. The blood film shows the presence of intracellular malaria parasites (*P. falciparum*). The parasites of *P. falciparum* are small (less than half the diameter of the red cell) and more than one may be seen in a red cell. Characteristically, they have a double chromatin dot. It is important not to confuse these with platelets over-lying red cells, an example of which is also shown in this field.

4. This shows the characteristic cells seen in glandular fever. These cells are large with abundant pale blue cytoplasm which invaginates itself round the red cells. These cells are not monocytes but T lymphocytes. The diagnosis may be confirmed by demonstrating antibodies to Epstein-Barr virus. Classically, this is done by the Paul-Bunnel test in which 'heterophil' antibodies are detected using sheep red cells. A similar picture may be seen with infection due to cytomegalovirus (CMV).

5. This is an LE cell. This is an *in vitro* phenomenon demonstrated by incubating the patient's serum with normal control blood. The LE cell is a neutrophil which has ingested nuclear debris. Although specific for systemic lupus erythematosus, it has low sensitivity and has largely been superseded by demonstration of antibodies against double stranded DNA.

6. There are microspherocytes on the blood film. The likely diagnosis is hereditary spherocytosis which can be confirmed by showing increased osmotic fragility. Hereditary spherocytosis is frequently demonstrated in several generations of the same family. The number of microspherocytes on the blood film may be relatively low prior to splenectomy and may be missed on casual examination. An additional feature may be the occurrence of jaundice in the neonatal period. The main differential diagnosis is auto-immune haemolytic anaemia. A negative direct antiglobulin test (direct Coomb's test) is more in keeping with hereditary spherocytosis.

7. Five plasma cells are demonstrated and the likely diagnosis is multiple myeloma. In this disorder, the marrow plasma cells are increased in number and are frequently found in clumps of 4 to 20. In extreme cases, sheets of plasma cells may be seen. The plasma cells have a typically abundant basophilic cytoplasm with a perinuclear clear zone representing the Golgi complex. The eccentric nucleus has clumped, peripheral chromatin (so-called clock face nucleus). The diagnosis can be confirmed by demonstrating a paraprotein in the serum or urine with osteolytic lesions on x-ray of the skeleton.

8. This is acute graft-versus-host disease (GVHD). Although the skin biopsy may be relatively non-specific, lymphocytic infiltration with necrosis of individual epidermal cells often leaves a characteristic clear area (so-called drop out phenomenon).

9. These red cells are acanthocytes. These may be seen in conjunction with abetalipoproteinaemia or acquired in relation to severe liver disease. Acanthocytes are one of a number of abnormal red cells characterised by the presence of spicules. Acanthocyte spicules are tall, pointed and narrow and their number is relatively low (fewer than 10 per cell). Some distortion of the cell may be seen. Acanthocytes are sometimes called spur cells.

10. The likely diagnosis is essential thrombocythaemia, which is a myeloproliferative disorder. Morphologically, the marrow shows increased numbers of megakaryocytes. In this high-power field, several megakaryocytes are seen, some of which are uninuclear. In addition, the marrow shows increased cellularity with increases in both erythroid and myeloid elements.

11. The picture demonstrates regular areas of closely grouped purpura. The lesions are confined to the anterior part of the body. This is typical of self-induced purpura which is often produced by the technique of cupping. A characteristic feature is that the purpura are grouped in regular areas which are within easy reach of the hands.

12. The blasts are sudan black B positive which is characteristic of acute myeloid leukaemia. Cytochemistry in the
diagnosis of leukaemia has largely been superseded by
immunophenotyping techniques, the basis of which
depends on the demonstration of an antigen (usually on
the surface of the cell). The antigen is demonstrated by
its reaction with an antibody (which is usually monoclonal) which is shown by fluorescence of an attached
label. This can be done using conventional fluorescence
microscopy or by fluorescence activated cell sorter (FACS).

13. This is a leucoerythroblastic blood film showing both
normoblasts and early myeloid precursors. The causes
are marrow infiltration by tumour, myelofibrosis or,
occasionally seen in response to acute infection, severe
haemorrhage and haemolysis. The red-cell morphology
is relatively normal and would be more in keeping with
infiltration by tumour.

14. The blasts show localised dot positively which is
characteristic of cells of T lineage. In this case, this was
acute lymphoblastic leukaemia. These techniques have
been largely superseded by immunotyping which allows
more detailed subdivision of the leukaemia depending
on the lineage and degree of differentiation.

15. The marrow shows numerous blasts, a few promyelocytes and two mitotic figures. On the basis of this
morphology, it is difficult to differentiate between acute
myeloid leukaemia and acute lymphoblastic leukaemia.
Further investigations, including immunophenotyping,
cytochemistry and karyotypic analysis, will be required
to make final diagnosis. In fact, this was acute myeloid
leukaemia.

16. This marrow shows increased numbers of megakaryocytes suggesting premature platelet destruction. This is likely to be idiopathic thrombocytopenic purpura (ITP). The diagnosis can be confirmed by demonstrating increased amounts of platelet-associated surface immunoglobulin.

17. This is a tumour infiltration of the marrow showing the characteristic clumps of primitive cells which are of non-haemopoetic origin. These cells are typically seen in clumps and, more rarely, diffusely through the marrow.

18. A number of lymphocytes are demonstrated in this blood film with abundant cytoplasm, some of which has a rather wavy edge to it. This is hairy cell leukaemia. These cells show tartrate resistant acid phosphatase (TRAP) and are usually of B-cell lineage. The marrow often shows increased amounts of fibrous tissue which may account for the difficulty in marrow aspiration in these patients.

19. This is leishmaniasis (*L. donovanii*). This results in Kala-Azar which is characterised by massive splenomegaly and fever. Anaemia and leucopenia may also be present. The diagnosis may be made by finding leishmania in splenic or marrow puncture material.

20. A number of pale staining particles are seen in the blood film which are typical of cryoglobulin. Initial examination of the blood film suggested that the white cell count was normal but when the sample was warmed the white cell count was only 7.6 x 10^9/l. As the blood cools and the cryoglobin forms, the particles may be of

sufficient size to be counted by automated cell counters, either as white cells or as platelets. Spurious leucocytosis or thrombocytosis is a common presentation. In this case, the cryoglobin was type 1 and the underlying diagnosis was myeloma.

21. This shows diffuse, fine mottling typical of miliary tuberculosis. The patient has myelodysplastic syndrome. Atypical mycobacteria were found on examination of the trephine biopsy of the bone marrow.

22. The blood film shows a marked increase in small lymphocytes. The white cell count is greater than 100 x 10^9/l. The cells are small with a high nuclear cytoplasmic ratio and are typical of chronic lymphocytic leukaemia (CLL). In addition, a few smeared or basket cells can be seen which are also typical of this condition. In CLL, there is often a reduction in the immunoglobulins which may predispose to infection (the cause of death in about one third of these patients). Auto-immune haemolytic anaemia may also be seen.

23. This is a blood film from a patient with hereditary elliptocytosis. Unlike hereditary spherocytosis, this condition is rarely associated with significant haemolysis. The elliptocytes may be prominent (as shown), but other families may demonstrate only subtle elliptocytotic change. In some cases, the molecular basis is due to abnormalities of the spectrin molecule or, occasionally, of protein 4.1. In the majority of cases, hereditary elliptocytosis is inherited as an autosomal dominant condition.

24. The material shows typical apple green birefringence of amyloid when viewed under polarising light. The marrow is not the most frequent sight for primary amyloid involvement although it is worthwhile doing special stains when amyloid is suspected as it may obviate the need for other invasive procedures, e.g. rectal biopsy.

25. These cells with fine lacy intracellular material are reticulocytes. As red cells are released from the marrow, their amount of nucleic acid is high. These cells, when stained with usual May-Grunwald Giemsa stain, show as polychromatic cells. As the reticulocytes mature, the nucleic acids are broken down to soluble products by 5'-pyrimidine nucleotidase and then diffuse out of the cell. Using supravital stains, e.g. new methylene blue, the nucleic acid is seen as a fine lacy intracellular pattern. Reticulocytes are seen in increased numbers following acute blood loss, haematinic replacement and haemolysis.

26. The marrow demonstrates typical megaloblastic changes with the erythroid precursors showing typical nuclear cytoplasmic asynchrony which may be seen with B12 or folic deficiency. In addition, giant metamyelocytes and a hypersegmented neutrophil can be seen. Morphologically, it is impossible to distinguish between B12 and folic deficiency and, if urgent therapy is required because of the severe symptomatic anaemia, both haematinics should be given after obtaining blood samples for haematinic levels.

27. This is blast transformation of chronic granulocytic leukaemia (CGL), an almost invariable complication of this type of leukaemia. The median duration of CGL is approximately three years from the time of diagnosis. The

transformation, which may be either lymphoid (about 10%) or myeloid, is usually heralded by white cells becoming refractory to control with standard therapy. This results in a rapidly increasing white cell count and spleen size, and possibly some constitutional symptoms such as weight loss and night sweats. Additional chromosomal abnormalities are frequently found, the most common of which is the second Philadelphia chromosome. This may occur several months in advance of the morphological changes. Lymphoid transformation has a much better prognosis than myeloid transformation, and it may be possible to return the patient to the chronic phase. In myeloid transformation, even with aggressive chemotherapy, the chances of a patient returning to the chronic phrase are small (around 10%). Survival, after transformation, is around six months.

28. This demonstrates sickle cells from a patient with homozygous sickle cell anaemia.

29. This slide demonstrates sideroblasts. In a man of this age, the likely diagnosis is sideroblastic anaemia, which is classified as one of the myelodysplastic syndromes. This may occasionally (approximately 10% of cases) evolve to acute myeloid leukaemia. Other causes of acquired sideroblastic anaemia are often related to effects of drug therapy (including pyrazinamide) or chronic infection. Rarely, they may be seen as inherited disorders, usually autosomal dominant, some of which may be responsive to the use of high-dose pyridoxine (vitamin B6).

30. This is the hip and pelvic x-ray from a patient with sickle cell anaemia showing marked destruction of the right hip as a result of osteomyelitis. In sickle cell disease, this may be due to staphylococcal infection but a sizeable

minority of patients suffer from salmonella infection, which may result in chronic osteomyelitis and extensive bone destruction.

31. The film shows marrow comprising blast cells which have a high nuclear cytoplasmic ratio. In some of these cells, the nuclear chromatin is clumped while in others vacuolation can be seen. There is some variation in the size of the cells with a greater proportion of larger cells. Some of the cells show prominent nucleoli. The diagnosis is acute lymphoblastic leukaemia of FAB sub-type L2. This sub-type is more frequent in older age groups and some trials have shown it to carry a poorer prognosis than other FAB sub-types. The usual factors which determine prognosis are: age, white cell count at presentation, and sex.

32. The chest x-ray shows a number of opacities, particularly in the left lung fields. These are rounded and, in this context, are typical of aspergilloma. Indeed, this was confirmed at bronchoscopy. Treatment was with intravenous amphotericin.

33. The red cells are macrocytic and mostly round. A few target cells can also be seen. The small lymphocyte provides an idea of red-cell diameter, with most erythrocytes being larger than the diameter of the lymphocyte nucleus. The neutrophil is not hypersegmented which suggests liver disease, hypothyroidism or alcohol as the underlying cause (rather than B12 or folate deficiency). Cell size is difficult to gauge on peripheral blood films although, as above, the use of a lymphocyte nucleus to gauge size is helpful. However, most reliance would be placed on the mean cell volume (MCV) measured by modern electronic counters.

34. Anisocytosis (variation in size) of the red cells and several target cells can be seen. Several basophilic inclusions are also observed within the red cells (one of which contains two of these inclusion bodies). This typically occurs following splenectomy (which may be performed for a number of reasons). In addition, microspherocytes are often seen under these conditions although they may not be characteristic of the condition for which splenectomy was performed. Thrombocytosis and neutrophil leucocytosis are commonly seen after splenectomy although with time the number of platelets or neutrophils may return to normal.

35. In this blood film a large number of blasts cells are noted. The cells are quite pleomorphic: some have high nuclear cytoplasmic ratios and a number show binucleate forms. This is acute leukaemia and further investigation confirmed that this was of myeloid lineage and, in particular, FAB sub-type M5. Binucleate forms are typical of acute monocytic leukaemia.

36. The bands are seen running in the position of A and S. These are of equal intensity suggesting sickle cell trait. It would be important to know that the patient had not been transfused recently because it is possible to mimic sickle cell trait with transfusion in patients who are homozygous for HbS. It must be remembered that other haemoglobins migrate with the same mobility as HbS, e.g. HbD. These may be differentiated simply by performing the sickle solubility (sickledex) test or undertaking electrophoresis under different conditions, i.e. altered pH and media.

37. This shows the classical features of acute graft-versus-host disease (GVHD) with marked erythema and a macular rash which is often seen first on the palms and soles. Acute GVHD is due to the transplantation of immunocompetent lymphocytes with the donor graft which recognise HLA antigens on the skin. These produce an intense erythematous rash which may become confluent. Initially, this may be difficult to distinguish from a drug induced rash. However, the predilection to affect palms and soles strongly suggests GVHD. Skin biopsy may be helpful in clarification. The immunocompetent donor lymphocytes also recognise HLA antigens in the liver and gut and may affect these organs. Hepatocyte destruction may lead to hyperbilirubinaemia and other features of impaired hepatic function. GVHD affecting the gut usually presents with diarrhoea which is characteristically of large volume and watery.

38. The blood film shows the presence of atypical lymphocytes which have variable amounts of cytoplasm. In some cells, the cytoplasm shows marked border irregularity which gives rise to the common name of hairy cell leukaemia. Marrow fibrosis is common in this disorder and results in difficulty in marrow aspiration. The diagnosis can be confirmed either by cytochemistry or immunophenotyping. Treatment is usually by splenectomy, particularly if the spleen is bulky. Chemotherapy with either deoxycoformycin or interferon may also be used in the absence of splenomegaly, or if splenectomy has been ineffective.

39. A number of large, bizarre cells with abundant cytoplasm are illustrated, several of which show prominent vacuolation. The nuclei of the cells have open chromatin with multiple nuclei. This is acute leukaemia. The abundant cytoplasm and vacuolation would suggest a monocytic lineage which was indeed confirmed by further investigation. Gum infiltration is a common finding in mono-

cytic leukaemia but also occurs in other tissues, including the peritoneum, pericardium and pleura.

40. The arrowed chromosome (A) is an abnormal chromosome 22. It has resulted from the exchange of part of the long arm of chromosome 9 with the long arm of chromosome 22, resulting in a smaller than normal chromosome 22 (the Philadelphia chromosome) and larger chromosome 9 (B). The genetic material from chromosome 9 includes the abl gene which is translocated to a region in chromosome 22 known as the breakpoint cluster region (bcr). The fusion product (bcr-abl) produces a larger than normal protein which is the enzyme, tyrosine kinase. Philadelphia chromosome is seen in chronic granulocytic leukaemia and in a small number (10%) of patients with acute lymphoblastic leukaemia. In each condition, the bcr-abl fusion product has a different molecular size enabling precise diagnosis.

41. Fluorescence of several cells is noted, particularly neutrophil leucocytes. In addition, small specks of fluorescence are noted between the cells. This is due to the fluorescence of malarial parasites; in this case, falciparum malaria which was confirmed on conventionally stained blood film. This technique (Quantitative Buffy Coat. Becton Dickinson™) is an invaluable rapid screening method for the diagnosis of malaria — a one minute search being equivalent to a fifteen minute examination of conventional thick film.

42. In this film there is a large blast which has abundant and relatively agranular cytoplasm. However, there is a rod-like structure in the cytoplasm. This is an auer rod which is highly typical of acute myeloid leukaemia. The auer rod is formed by condensation of primary granules.

43. This blood film shows hypochromia, microcytosis and occasional target cells. The differential diagnosis would be iron deficiency anaemia and thalassaemia. Additional information may be obtained from measurement of serum ferritin. However, some people with ß- or α-thalassaemia also become iron deficient and ferritin may not always differentiate between these conditions. Correction of possible iron deficiency and repeat haemoglobin electrophoresis with demonstration of raised haemoglobin A2 may help. Red cell protoporphyrin assay may also be of value. In fact this is ß-thalassaemia trait.

44. The blood film shows an increase in the numbers of neutrophils and their precursors. In the area shown, several myelocytes are seen in addition to a blast. A basophil is seen at the edge of the field. An absolute increase in basophils was seen in this patient. In the marrow aspirate, marked hyperplasia of the myeloid series was noted in all stages of maturation including segmentation of neutrophils. However, there was a relative increase in the myelocytes which is characteristic of chronic granulocytic leukaemia (CGL). The diagnosis of chronic phase CGL was confirmed by the demonstration of the Philadelphia chromosome (see question 40). The major problem of CGL is transformation to acute leukaemia (see question 27), a development which is usually heralded by the acquisition of new chromosomal abnormalities.

45. This is an eosinophil. Eosinophils are the second most common of the granulocytes in peripheral blood which normally contains between 0.1–0.45 x 10^9/l. Eosinophils are slightly larger than neutrophils and have a bi-lobed nucleus. Their characteristic feature is the presence of granules which stain intensely with acid dyes such as eosin. The granules which appear early in maturation

contain a number of proteins, e.g. major basic protein, eosinophil cationic protein, eosinophil neurotoxin and peroxidase. The role of eosinophils appears to be in mediating immune response to helminthic infection, allergy and some tumours, e.g. Hodgkin's disease. Eosinophils respond to chemotactic factors and, although they may be capable of phagocytosis, their main function appears to be as a secretory cell. Secretion of a granule protein may cause damage (e.g. to helminths) or to tissues (e.g. endomyocardial fibrosis) as seen in hypereosinophilic syndromes.

46. This slide shows marked swelling of both knee joints which is particularly bad on the left side. In addition, wasting of the quadriceps is evident (again predominantly on the left side). This indicates that the process is chronic. In fact, this young man had haemophilia A and had experienced recurrent haemorrhages for many years. Unfortunately, he had developed an inhibitor to factor VIII which made the treatment of these haemorrhages more difficult.

47. Several lumps are noted on the skin. These vary in size and generally have a blueish tint to them. One has already been biopsied. The biopsy showed infiltration by primitive myeloid cells confirming the clinical diagnosis of leukaemia cutis. The blood film at this point showed an increasing number of myeloid blasts. The transformation of polycythaemia rubra vera to acute leukaemia is well recognised, although a relatively rare occurrence.

48. There are a number of neutrophils with enhanced granulation. This is toxic granulation. In addition, some of the neutrophils show pale basophilic inclusion bodies.

These are Döhle bodies and are typical of neutrophils seen in patients with severe acute infections or burns (particularly children with severe infection).

49. The blood film shows round macrocytosis, and neutrophil leucocytes with vacuolation. The combination of these two features is highly suggestive of ethanol effects on the bone marrow. Ethanol will affect all three cell lines, although its principal effects are seen in red-cell production (with marrow erythroblasts showing vacuolation and mature red cells being often larger than normal). Impaired neutrophil and platelet production are common features. Target cells are frequent. As illustrated, the neutrophils show vacuolation and may exhibit a functional defect.

50. The blood film shows increased numbers of nucleated red cells and polychromatic erythrocytes. In addition, some spherocytes are also seen. This, together with the jaundice, is typical of haemolytic disease of the newborn (HDN) which is due to the transplacental passage of antibodies directed against red cell antigens. The most important antibody is directed against the rhesus D antigen but antibodies to other rhesus and red-cell antigens, e.g. Kell, are all associated with severe HDN. The diagnosis can be confirmed by a positive direct Coombs test on cord cells and demonstrating the presence of an antibody directed against foetal red cells in the mother.

51. The blood film shows a marked increase in platelets with numerous large or giant platelets, some of which are almost as big as red cells. The platelet count was $850 \times 10^9/l$. The bone marrow was hypercellular, with increased numbers of megakaryocytes, and shows

increased amounts of reticulin which confirmed the diagnosis of essential thrombocythaemia.

52. Most of the red cells are small and poorly haemo-globinised, i.e. the cells show hypochromia and micro-cytosis. The size of the cells can be gauged against the small lymphocyte shown (normal red cells should be slightly larger than the diameter of the small lymphocyte). In this film, most of the cells are considerably smaller. The area of central pallor is also increased. The likely diag-nosis is iron deficiency anaemia but thalassaemia and anaemia of chronic disorder should also be considered.

53. The striking feature is the presence of microspherocytes. These are small cells which stain more intensely red than normal cells. In addition, there is a nucleated red cell and a number of larger cells which have a blue tinge. With a supravital stain, e.g. new methylene blue, these would be seen as reticulocytes. The number of neutrophils is also increased suggesting infection. This patient had an acute haemolytic crisis with hereditary spherocytosis associated with infection. The Direct Coomb's test was negative. The diagnosis could be confirmed with osmotic fragility studies in both the patient and other members of the family.

54. Numerous red cell fragments are shown in this film with some polychromasia which is suggestive of micro-angiopathic haemolytic anaemia. The most important disorders associated with this are haemolytic uraemia syndrome (HUS), thrombotic thrombocytopenic purpura (TTP), eclampsia, malignant hypertension and disseminated intravascular coagulopathy (DIC). The cause of the red-cell changes is due to the deposition of fibrin in small vessels, i.e. arterioles, particularly in the kidney. The pathophysiology may vary in different dis-orders, e.g. in TTP but not in HUS very high molecular weight multimers of von Willebrand factor are seen.

55. Numerous microspherocytes are seen in this blood film. In addition, some of the cells show, usually single, basophilic inclusions. These are Howell-Jolly bodies and are seen following splenectomy. The direct antiglobulin test was positive. Diagnosis is auto-immune haemolytic anaemia which had been present for many years. Steroids had not been particularly effective and the patient had a splenectomy to control the haemolysis with some effect.

56. Large numbers of blast cells are seen. There is some pleomorphism but most of the cells show a high nuclear cytoplasmic ratio and generally open nuclei chromatin with large nuclei. Further investigation confirmed this to be acute myeloid leukaemia of FAB sub-type M5.

57. The blood film shows the presence of malaria parasites. In this case the parasites are *P. vivax* (see question 3).

58. The marrow shows the presence of numerous blast cells which are pleomorphic, some larger cells are also noted. Most of the blasts have prominent nuclei. Further investigation showed these cells to be sudan black positive and positive for non-specific and chloroacetate esterase. These cytochemical reactions are typical of acute myelomonocytic leukaemia which could be further confirmed by marking the surface membrane with appropriate monoclonal antibodies, e.g. CD14, CD33.

59. This shows an abnormal granulocyte precursor which has abundant cytoplasm showing marked granularity. The nucleus is eccentric in position, has a nucleolus and, in some cases, shows a slight indentation. These features are typical of acute promyelocytic leukaemia. One of

the features of this disorder is the frequent occurrence of bleeding problems due to disseminated intravascular coagulation (DIC). This is initiated by the release of pro-coagulant material from the blasts and promyelocytes resulting in activation of clotting mechanism and consumption of clotting factors. DIC may be precipitated by the start of cytoreductive chemotherapy. The use of the differentiating agent all-trans-retinoic acid (ATRA) may prevent this potentially fatal complication. Acute promyelocytic leukaemia is associated with a characteristic chromosomal translocation involving chromosomes 15 and 17 (t 15, 17).

60. The red cells show infestation with *P. malariae*. This form of malaria, which causes quartan malaria, is probably the least common seen in this region. The infestation is usually slight, with fewer than 1% of red cells being infected — emphasising the care required in examining the blood film. The red cell is usually not enlarged (unlike *P.ovale* infestation) and shizonts are small and compact. It may be difficult to distinguish from ovale malaria except that in the latter the host red cell is usually oval or irregular in shape (see questions 3 and 57).

61. The red cells are microcytic (small) and poorly haemo-globinised (hypochromic). There are some target cells. The differential diagnosis is iron deficiency and thalass-aemia, although in other clinical situations, e.g. rheuma-toid arthritis, anaemia of chronic disorder might also produce a similar picture. For the same haemo-globin concentration the mean corpuscular volume (MCV) is lower in thalassaemia than in the other two conditions and this is used in several discriminant functions based on red-cell indices which may help to distinguish these conditions. Ultimately, the distinction rests on the demonstration of a raised haemoglobin A2 in ß-thalassaemia and low serum ferritin in iron deficiency.

62. The blood film shows an increased number of white cells. These cells have a very high nuclear cytoplasmic ratio with some clumping of the chromatin and generally single nucleoli. At this age, the likely diagnosis is that of acute lymphoblastic leukaemia (ALL). In this case, markers were positive for CD10, i.e common ALL. The blast cell count was high at $40 \times 10^9/l$ which, together with the sex of the patient, is a poor prognostic feature. However, age is favourable. Treatment would be with standard regimes involving the use of prednisolone, vincristine and adriamycin as initial induction therapy.

63. The white cell shown is a large lymphocyte with few azurophilic granules in the cytoplasm. This is a large granular lymphocyte (LGL), an increase in which is often associated with splenomegaly and neutropenia in a condition known as large granular lymphocytic leukaemia. LGLs show the immunophenotype of natural killer cells (CD3 positive, CD8 positive, CD16 positive). In the original reported series, about 50% of the cases were associated with sero-positive rheumatoid arthritis. Doubt ensued whether this condition was truly neoplastic and not merely a reactive phenomenon. However, demonstration of rearrangement of the T-cell receptor genes have confirmed the clonal nature of this disorder. It is usually benign with the neutropenia being easily reversed with steroid therapy, when necessary.

64. This is a Pelger neutrophil. This cell is typically seen in myelodysplastic syndromes. The cell has a bi-lobed nucleus with a thin chromatin bridge between the lobes. This appearance has sometimes been likened to pince nez spectacles. The cytoplasm is hypogranular. This is also a rarely reported congenital anomaly.

65. The blood film shows marked variation in the size of the red cells. In addition, fragmented red cells can be seen, some of which show a characteristic helmet appearance. Several blister cells are also observed. In these cells, it appears as if the red cell membrane has lifted off from the underlying haemoglobin, giving the appearance of a blister on the skin. These changes are characteristic of G6PD deficiency. The diagnosis could be confirmed by assaying for this enzyme, although care must be taken with interpretation in the presence of a raised reticulocyte count, which is associated with elevated enzyme activity. In G6PD deficiency, haemolysis is usually precipitated by exposure to oxidising agents, including drugs such as sulphonamides.

66. The blood film shows rouleaux. These red cells appear to be stacked one on top of the other rather like a column of coins which has been pushed over on its side. It is usually associated with a high ESR and may be seen in any infective or inflammatory cause. It is also commonly seen in myeloma. However, in situations when there is a paraprotein, a clue is often given by the presence of background basophilic staining due to the high level of plasma protein.

67. With the MGG stain, the marrow shows a cluster of non-haemopoetic cells which are rather pleomorphic, but show a clear area around the nucleus suggestive of carcinoma. The cells are also PAS positive and probably have their origin in the gastrointestinal tract.

68. This is a hypersegmented neutrophil. In this case, the neutrophil shows eight or nine separate lobes and is, in fact, of larger size than normal. The surrounding red

cells are also larger. This would be typical of a hyper-segmented neutrophil seen in either B12 or folic acid deficiency.

69. The marrow shows a macrophage which is heavily laden with blue staining material. This material is haemosiderin and is suggestive of iron overload which is usually associated with transfusion. It is unusual to see a great increase in haemosiderin laden macrophages in haemochromatosis. However, this latter diagnosis should be considered and, if necessary, can be confirmed by liver biopsy and family studies. It is important to distinguish this cell from ringed sideroblasts seen in sideroblastic anaemia.

70. In this area of the aspirate, there is an increase in the number of small lymphocytes accounting for approximately 30% of the total. The lymphocytes show some plasmacytoid differentiation with chromatin clumping into the typical clock face. However, the typical plasma cells are not seen in this example. In some cases of Waldenstrom's macroglobulinaemia the typical infiltrate of lymphocytes and plasma cells may not always be seen. In fact in this case, the trephine biopsy, a more typical mixed appearance was noted. This should be contrasted with question number 34.

71. The blood shows marked increase in the number of nucleated red cells. In addition, the non-nucleated red cells are small and purely haemoglobinised. Increased numbers of target cells are also noted. The haemoglobin was only 7.3 g/dl and the likely diagnosis is ß-thalassaemia intermedia. The diagnosis could be confirmed by measuring HbA2 and by family studies.

72. These red cells are target cells. Normal red cells have an area of central pallor while target cells show an area of central haemoglobinisation. Target cells are thought to be produced in situations when there is an imbalance in the ratio of the amounts of red-cell membrane and haemoglobin, i.e. excess membrane or decreased amounts of haemoglobin. Situations where this is seen include liver disease in which, due to derangement in fat metabolism, there is thought to be an accumulation of membrane after the red cell is released from the marrow. These target cells are large, i.e. macrocytic, although in situations where there is poor haemoglobinisation (classically seen in thalassaemia or in some haemo-globinopathies, e.g. HbC) they are small. In these situations, the red cell produces this complex arrangement with central areas of haemoglobin instead of forming the normal biconcave disc. Target cells are also known as Mexican hat cells.

73. The striking feature is the presence of a myeloblast with a high nuclear cytoplasmic ratio and several prominent nucleoli. Numerous similar cells were seen in the peripheral blood and the marrow. The diagnosis was transformation to acute myeloblastic leukaemia (AML). There is an increased incidence of AML in polycythaemia rubra vera. As a result of the possible increased risk of leukaemia following radio-active phosphorus exposure, current treatment with hydroxyurea would be the preferred option, particularly in the younger patient. The more usual course in polycythaemia rubra vera is transformation to myelo-fibrosis. This results in increasing splenomegaly (which may alone cause symptoms) and increasing anaemia, which may result in the patient becoming red cell transfusion dependant.

74. The marrow shows prominent macrophages, many of which are showing haemophagocytosis (see macrophage in the centre of the field). In adults, this is usually seen as a reactive phenomenon, particularly to viral infections (e.g. hepatitis, HIV 1) and tuberculosis. It may also be seen as a primary phenomenon in histiocytic medullary reticulosis, although in this case some authorities believe that the macrophages which appear to be malignant often fail to show haemophagocytosis. This woman, who was from the Indian subcontinent, was subsequently shown (by culture of bronchioli washings) to have mycobacterium tuberculosis. In this situation, the diagnosis had been suggested and she was able to start anti-tuberculosis therapy before the arrival of the culture results.

75. The blood film shows red cells with coarse basophilic stippling. This may occur as an artefact arising from the stain pH being too low or, alternatively, may be seen in congenital deficiency of pyrimidine 5'-nucleotidase (an enzyme responsible for breaking down pyrimidine nucleotides which are breakdown products of RNA). Basophilic stippling is also seen in lead poisoning which, in view of the history of abdominal pain, is the likely diagnosis. Lead poisoning can be confirmed either by measuring plasma lead levels or, more easily, by measuring erythrocyte protoporphyrin level, which is raised enormously under these circumstances. Although previously found in children who ingested lead from lead-based paints, it is now usually seen as a result of industrial exposure to lead oxide paints (which were commonly used to rustproof steel) or in workers dealing with old car batteries.

76. There is a large medial swelling over the lower third of the left thigh. The man wears a support bandage on his right knee but muscle wasting of the quadriceps is

apparent, particularly over the medial aspect. The likely diagnosis is a left-sided muscle haematoma and right-sided haemarthrosis in a patient with haemophilia, probably due to factor VIII C, i.e. haemophilia A. Treatment should consist of the replacement of factor VIII C using suitable concentrate (aiming to bring factor VIII C level to around 30–40% of normal). This would be continued twice daily for several days until the bleeding has settled. In addition, general measures, e.g. adequate pain control, physiotherapy and support for the knee, would be required during recovery phase. Prophylactic treatment with factor VIII C would be likely to prevent future recurrence.

77. The blood film shows an absence of platelets, i.e. thrombocytopenia. This serves to differentiate between the 'vascular' purpuras, such as Henoch-Schonlein, and 'thrombocytopenia' purpura. The likeliest cause of thrombocytopenia in a child of this age is due to immune destruction of platelets (i.e. ITP) although other causes, including failure of production of platelets (e.g. congenital amegakaryocytopoiesis, Fanconi syndrome, aplastic anaemia and leukaemia), need to be considered. Disseminated intravascular coagulopathy is also an important cause of premature platelet destruction. Careful examination of the blood film and marrow aspirate/trephine will allow differentiation between the causes. Presence of leukaemic blasts or aplasia will be shown. ITP can be confirmed by demonstrating increased platelet surface immunoglobulins but should not be considered a diagnosis itself but a sign of a secondary cause, e.g. lymphoma or systemic lupus erythematosus.

78. The patient shows an increase in osmotic fragility with mean cell fragility (MCF) of 0.54g NaCl/l. This is characteristic of spherocytosis and indeed the patient had

microspherocytes on blood film. Several family members were also affected. In some patients, the osmotic fragility using fresh blood is normal but it becomes abnormal following incubation of red cells for 24 hours.

79. The x-ray shows widening of the upper mediastinum and prominant hilar lymphadenopathy. The likely diagnosis is Hodgkin's disease or non-Hodgkin's lymphoma. Sarcoid might also be considered. The diagnosis could be confirmed by biopsy of the cervical lymph node.

80. The marrow shows marked erythroid hyperplasia. Many of the normoblasts are suggestive of a congenital dyserythropoeitic anaemia. Of the three recognised types of this disorder, type 1 is characterised by chromosome bridges between the nuclei of the erythroblasts. Type 3 is characterised by large multi-nucleated normoblasts and the observation that the mature red cells are readily agglutinated by antibodies. Type 2 is the most common and is characterised by a positive reaction to Ham's test, i.e. the cells show increased susceptibility to haemolysis in acidified serum. The cells are usually binucleate in the marrow, although occasionally the trinucleate form is seen. A double nuclear membrane is seen on electron microscopy.

81. There is obvious swelling of the neck and pre-auricular areas. The likely diagnosis is lymphoma. Further investigation should initially include excision of the node for histological examination, CT scans of head, neck, chest, abdomen and pelvis to detect further lymphadenopathy, and bone marrow examination.

82. The striking feature of this slide is the marked pallor of one of the twins who also appears smaller with plethera of the other twin. This is characteristic of twin-to-twin transfusion.

83. The normal marrow architecture is largely disrupted with some areas of bluish staining and fibrin-like material replacing some of the marrow cells. The marrow cells themselves, some of which look quite indistinct, probably represent necrotic cells. This is typical of bone marrow necrosis. This may be seen in association with acute leukaemia, particularly acute lymphoblastic leukaemia or sickle cell anaemia.

84. The head, neck and upper body of a middle-aged man are shown. Some bruising of the anterior chest is noted and the hands and face look plethoric. There is suggestion of cervical adenopathy. The diagnosis is superior vena caval obstruction, probably secondary to lymphoma affecting the drainage through the superior vena caval system.

85. This demonstrates Heinz bodies. These are due to denatured oxidised haemoglobin and are found in G6PD deficiency and also unstable haemoglobins. This type of anaemia is associated with bite cells, which are also seen on the blood film. Heinz bodies are not seen with usual stains, e.g. Wright's or May-Grunwald Giemsa.

86. There is a florid maculopapular rash of bluish colour over the upper part of the body. Some of these papules are almost nodular in appearance and are suggestive of an infiltrate. Taken in the context of the history, this is very suggestive of adult T-cell leukaemia lymphoma

(ATLL) which is associated with HTLV1 virus infection. This virus is endemic in parts of the West Indies, Africa and Japan. It is associated with the development of both ATLL and spastic paraparesis.

87. Large numbers of teardrop poikilocytes are shown on this blood film. These cells are usually seen in myelo-fibrosis, but also occur with megaloblastic anaemia. However, the presence of massive splenomegaly would be more in keeping with the former diagnosis. Frequently, immature red cell and white cell precursors are seen due to the presence of extra-medullary haemopoiesis.

88. This shows the presence of large blasts with a high nuclear cytoplasmic ratio and basophilic cytoplasm. There are no granules. The chromatin has a very open appearance with most of the cells showing large nuclei which tend to be seen at their periphery. These are characteristic of erythroblasts and indeed this is erythro-leukaemia. This is a rare form of leukaemia. It is almost certainly a secondary leukaemia arising against a background of pre-existing myelodysplastic syndrome. A mixture of erythroid and myeloid blasts is often present. The erythroid blasts characteristically show marked positivity with the PAS stain.

89. There is a purpuric rash on the lower legs which is particularly noticeable around hair follicles. This is characteristic of scurvy due to vitamin C deficiency.

90. This shows telangiectasia. This is often seen as a familial condition which presents with recurrent bleeding from the upper gastrointestinal tract and the nose, resulting in severe iron deficiency anaemia. These patients are often transfused on a regular basis because of the anaemia.

91. There is marked blue-yellow discolouration of the basal ganglia. This is a classic appearance of kernicterus arising from high levels of unconjugated bilirubin in the neonatal period. This is most often due to haemolytic disease of the newborn which should be treated with exchange transfusion before secondary brain damage occurs.

92. This shows marked differentiation between the cortex and medulla with depression of the end plate of the vertebral body. This is characteristic of a sickle cell disease and is due to necrosis of the vertebral growth plates. The outer portion of the growth plates are spared resulting in this characteristic deformity in which the depressions are confined to the central portion. This gives an appearance which has been described as similar to a fishmouth.

93. Large numbers of blast cells are noted. The blasts are quite pleomorphic and some very large cells with abundant bluish cytoplasm can be seen. Other cells are quite small with a high nuclear cytoplasmic ratio. Most of the cells have prominent nuclei. The cytoplasm is featureless. The appearances are compatible with acute myeloid leukaemia. Further cytochemical staining confirmed the impression of monocytic component, i.e. acute myelomonocytic leukaemia.

94. There is an area of necrosis and erythema stretching over the antecubital fossa. Extravasation of chemotherapy which has been given by IV infusion through a cannula in one of the antecubital veins has caused necrosis of skin and subcutaneous tissues. This is a very serious complication and may result in considerable morbidity. It illustrates the importance of having secure venous excess when giving chemotherapy.

95. There is an extensive rash and erythema over the back and arms of this patient. Hyperpigmentation and areas of thickening, particularly over the flexors can be seen. These appearances are highly suggestive of graft-versus-host disease.

96. There is intense erythema of the hands and face and, in fact, of the whole body of this woman. This is erythroderma associated with Hodgkin's disease — a rare complication of this disorder. It is not due to skin infiltration, but is presumably related to cytokines released from Hodgkin's cells.

97. The x-ray shows numerous lytic lesions, particularly in the lower third of the femur. These are suggestive of myeloma which can be confirmed by finding a malignant paraprotein in the serum or urine together with an absolute plasmacytosis in the bone marrow.

98. This is a pack of whole blood which is group O, rhesus negative. Group O rhesus-negative blood is traditionally known as universal donor blood. This is suitable for use in emergencies as it can be used uncrossmatched when there is insufficient time to await the arrival of

homologous group checked blood of appropriate ABO and rhesus grouping. This practice is not, however, without problems. The presence of high-titre anti A or B in group O donors has been associated with severe haemolytic reactions and even death. It is important that before these units are made available for use in this way that they are checked to ensure that there are no dangerous haemolysins present.

99. This shows an eruption on the left side of the chest. The eruption appears to be vesicular although some of the vesicles appear to have become haemorrhagic. It is localised to one dermatome, probably T8. This is herpes zoster or shingles. For most patients this is a self-limiting, if rather painful, condition. However, in immunosuppressed patients, for example, those with acute leukaemia or lymphoma, infection with herpes zoster can result in disseminated spread and therefore demands early treatment. The diagnosis can be confirmed rapidly by electron microscopy of the vesicular fluid and treatment commenced using acyclovir (either alone or in association with specific immunoglobin directed against the virus).

100. This shows a typical cyst of toxoplasma. Toxoplasma infection may be associated with lymphadenopathy; it is important in the evaluation of any patient with unexplained lymphadenopathy that toxoplasma serology is checked.

101. This shows two vials of human factor IX concentrate which is used in the replacement therapy of haemophilia B. This is an intermediate purity product which also contains factors II and X. Concentrate of this kind, prepared by ethanol fractionation, has been associated with

thrombotic episodes, particularly when large doses have been given — for example, to cover surgical procedures in patients with haemophilia B.

102. Necrosis of the ends of the fingers of the right hand is shown in this patient. This was associated with the presence of a cold agglutinin. In this case, the necrosis occurred after exposure to cold with the agglutination of red cells resulting in stasis and consequential hypoxia, producing necrosis of the finger tips. Cold agglutinins may be associated with an underlying lymphoma although occasionally no cause may be found. A similar picture can be caused by cryoglobulins.

103. This series of CT scans shows infarction in the posterior poles of the occipital cortex. This is extended anteriorly to affect the parietal lobes. Cerebral infarction is more common in children with sickle cell disease. It is clearly of major importance and may result in considerable mobidity. Recurrence may be prevented by establishing these patients on a transfusion regime to reduce their HbS to around 30% of normal. Although there is no clear evidence how long this should be continued, at least five years seems appropriate.

104. This shows a flat-bed platelet agitator with a unit of platelet concentrate. Continuous agitation at room temperature maximises the storage time of platelets. Platelet concentrate should be used for patients with severe thrombocytopenia who are bleeding or in those with platelet counts below 15 to 20 x $10^9/l$ as a prophylactic measure.

105. This shows hyperplastic bleeding and probably infected gums. This may be seen in acute leukaemia but is also a feature of scurvy (which is associated with a normal full blood count). In this situation, careful examination of the skin may well reveal the typical peripheral purpura and hair changes associated with scurvy. This condition is rapidly reversible with the introduction of vitamin C.

106. The skull x-ray shows multiple osteolytic lesions which, when in the skull, are usually associated with multiple myeloma. However, this condition is excessively rare in people under 30 years of age. This diagnosis was a high-grade non-Hodgkin's lymphoma.

107. This shows the sickle solubility (sickledex) test. This consists of dropping a few drops of blood into a specific buffer with a reducing agent in which HbS is insoluble and therefore precipitates making it impossible to read the chart behind the test tube. Normal haemoglobin remains soluble as do other variants. This test, therefore, only detects the presence of HbS and does not indicate the phenotype of the patient.

108. The chest x-ray shows bilateral basal shadowing, which is possibly worse on the right. The differential diagnosis is pneumonic consolidation or sickle chest syndrome although it is difficult radiologically to distinguish between the two. Unilateral signs would be more in keeping with chest infection, although this is not absolute. Similarly, sickle cell chest syndrome is usually associated with greater degrees of hypoxia although this may also fail to be entirely discriminatory. In these situations, it is advisable to manage the patient as if it

were acute chest syndrome with urgent exchange blood transfusion aiming to bring the HbS percentage to around 30%. This may require several manual exchange transfusions in addition to the usual supportive therapies, including rehydration, oxygen and antibiotics.

109. This shows the presence of some perifollicular purpura and hairs which have a characteristic corkscrew appearance. This is typical of scurvy due to vitamin C deficiency.

110. There is obvious bleeding from the gums which are clearly hypertrophied. The differential diagnosis should include acute leukaemia, scurvy and other bleeding problems. A full blood count and blood film should be helpful in this situation. In acute leukaemia, anaemia and thrombocytopenia are almost invariable while the white cell count may be either low, normal or high. Examination of the blood film will reveal the presence of abnormal blast cells suggestive of acute myeloid leukaemia, particularly its monocytic variants.

111. There is a very obvious abnormality of the circulation on the right arteriogram. The kidney appears to be displaced slightly downwards suggesting a tumour. The resected kidney shows a large tumour occupying the upper pole of the kidney. Histological examination showed this to be a renal carcinoma. These tumours may secrete erythropoietin which stimulates the marrow to produce red cells, producing a secondary polycythaemia. In investigating a patient with polycythaemia two questions have to be answered. The first is to determine whether this is true or pseudo-polycythaemia. The second is whether the true polycythaemia is primary or secondary. The first question can be answered by red-cell volume studies which will show if the high haemo-

globin is due to an increase in red-cell mass or a decreased plasma volume. The secondary polycythaemias are more difficult to delineate. Some features may suggest primary polycythaemia, e.g. raised white cell count, raised platelet count, splenomegaly, raised serum B12, raised uric acid and raised leucocyte alkaline phosphatase (LAP) score. However, in the absence of these, the possibility of secondary polycythaemia exists. Careful clinical examination may show the presence of a congenital heart defect but further investigation should include pulmonary function studies with measurement of arterial blood gases (including carboxyhaemoglobin) which will delineate secondary polycythaemia due to respiratory causes. Thereafter, ultrasound or CT scan of the abdomen should be performed to establish the presence of renal lesions, hepatic carcinomas or cysts. A CT scan of the head should be similarly performed to exclude cerebellar haemangiomata.

112. The red-cell life span is around 120 days. It is possible to label a cohort of red cells using either ^{14}C-glycine or ^{59}Fe and follow its survival. However, these techniques are time consuming, laborious and probably not very satisfactory. The more usual method involves random labelling, using either ^{51}Cr or ^{32}P, of a group of red cells. These cells are then re-injected and the disappearance of the labelled cells is measured over the next two to three weeks. Using ^{51}Cr, the half-life of the labelled red cells has a normal range of 25–35 days. In this case, the half-life is around six days. The mean life span can be estimated by extrapolating the line to where it cuts the abscissa. However, in some cases the plot on arithmetic graph paper results in a line which is not straight. As in the case shown, the solution is to plot the values on semilogarithmic paper. Here the red cell life span is the time at which 37% of the cells are still surviving which, in this case, is around 10 days. Red-cell survival studies are often undertaken to determine the cause of anaemia when haemolysis and blood loss may be occurring in the same patient. It is useful to combine red-cell survival with a gastrointestinal (GI) blood loss study (involving a five-day collection of faeces) by measuring any radioactivity in the faeces to give an accurate measure of GI blood loss. This result can be used to recalculate the mean red-cell life span.

113. This illustration shows bottles of factor VIII concentrate 8Y, an intermediate purity concentrate, and 8SM, a monoclonal purified concentrate. Both are used in the treatment of haemophilia A to replace the deficient factor VIII. Factor VIII concentrates undergo a viral inactivation procedure. There is probably little to choose between intermediate and high-purity concentrates in terms of efficacy. However, there is no doubt that in patients who are HIV positive the purer concentrate, i.e. monoclonally purified, is associated with a slower decline in the number of CD4 positive lymphocytes. However, the highly purified products appear to contain less von Willebrands factor and are not, therefore, recommended for use in von Willebrands disease when an alternative source (for example, intermediate purity factor VIII or specific von Willebrand factor) must be used.

114. This is a bottle of factor IX concentrate which has been prepared using a monoclonal purification procedure and, as such, contains virtually pure factor IX. The older concentrates (the so-called prothrombin complex concentrates) were a mixture of factor IX plus factor II and factor X. For many years, these were the mainstay of treatment in haemophilia B (Christmas disease). However, their use was associated with an increased risk of thrombosis, perhaps related to the very high levels of factor II and factor X, which was seen after post-surgical replacement. Concentrate activation may also have played a role and many of these contained heparin to prevent this.

115. This is a bleeding time device (Simplate™). The device consists of a spring-loaded blade which, when released, results in a standard incision. The bleeding time is highly dependent upon the platelet count and platelet function and is therefore abnormal in thrombocytopenia, platelet functional defects (particularly when associated with aspirin) and von Willebrands disease. It tends to be normal in plasma defects of haemostasis.

116. This is a palmar erythema due to cytosine arabinoside treatment. It is a relatively rare complication which is seen as erythema of the palms and soles starting four or five days after chemotherapy has been given. Ultimately, desquamation of the surface epidermis occurs.

117. There is virtually no marrow seen in this trephine with the overall cellularity being about 10%. Most of the marrow spaces are replaced by fat. This is typical of aplastic anaemia.

118. There is a large amount of reticulin deposition showing large thick branching strands, some of which are coalescing to form thick strands. There appears to be a relationship between these strands and the megakaryocytes. The appearances are typical of myelofibrosis.

119. This shows an example of proliferative retinopathy in a patient with HbSC disease. The eye may also be involved in a number of additional complications including orbital infarction. Peripheral arteriolar occlusion may be one of the earliest changes which eventually progresses through to neovascularisation, haemorrhage and retinal detachment. Early opthalmic screening is needed

to detect these changes and, in a few cases, initiate photocoagulation therapy which may prevent progression to proliferative stages and blindness. Sickle cell retinopathy is seen more frequently in HbSC disease than homozygous sickle cell disease (HbSS).

120. The blood film shows many target cells. This is typical of HbC either in the homozygous or heterozygous state or in compound heterozygous states such as with HbS. Occasionally crystals of HbC can be seen within the red cells.

121. Several cells showing irregular blue-staining inclusions are seen. Inclusions are regularly spaced throughout the cell giving an appearance of a golf ball. These are HbH inclusions. HbH is a tetramer of ß-globin.

122. There is obvious enlargement of the left hilum almost certainly due to lymphadenopathy. There is some suggestion of consolidation extending to the left upper zone. There is no other lymphadenopathy and no tracheal deviation. The appearances are suggestive of lymphoma although it is impossible to distinguish between Hodgkin's disease and non-Hodgkin's disease radiologically. Clinical examination will reveal whether there is lymphadenopathy or organomegaly in other areas. CT scan will delineate the extent of the lymphadenopathy, if any, in other areas inaccessible to palpation. Diagnosis will depend on biopsy of a suitable node.

123. A number of lytic lesions are seen in the skull which are typical of myeloma, although (as seen in question 106) not all lytic lesions may result from this. The possibility of another lymphoma should always be borne in mind.

124. The hilar lymph nodes are enlarged, which is highly suggestive of their involvement. If further staging procedures show the disease to be confined above the diaphragm, it may be possible to treat it using radiotherapy alone. Nodular sclerosing disease, however, (where there may be bulky mediastinal involvement) is probably best treated with both chemotherapy and radiotherapy at the sites of bulky disease.

125. This fetus, which was stillborn, shows marked swelling of the tissues with enlargement of the liver and spleen. This is typical of hydropic fetus. From a haematological view point, the two important causes are severe haemolytic disease (usually due to rhesus incompatibility between mother and fetus) and severe α-thalassaemia (with no α chain production) resulting in haemoglobin Barts and severe intrauterine anaemia.

126. A number of gallstones are demonstrated within the gall bladder and the cause of the pain is cholecystitis. Typical bone changes of sickle cell disease are seen, particularly in the vertebral bodies. A large number of patients with congenital chronic haemolytic states, such as sickle cell disease, develop gallstones particularly in their second and third decades. It is probably worthwhile performing a routine ultrasound scan of the gall bladder and, if gallstones are present, elective cholecystectomy should be considered.

127. This shows a lead line which is seen as a faint blue line just below the gingival margins. It is usually associated with lead poisoning which characteristically gives basophilic stippling on the blood film.

128. This is a neutrophil which is the most common of the white cells in the peripheral blood in adulthood, although in childhood they are less frequent. They are actively phagocytic and are particularly important in bacterial infection.

129. This is a normal small lymphocyte. The nucleus of these cells are slightly smaller than normal red cells and can be used to determine the size of the latter, albeit in an approximate manner. The small lymphocyte has a high nuclear cytoplasmic ratio and only a small rim of agranular cytoplasm is seen.

130. This cell is a monocyte. It is the largest of the white cells in peripheral blood and has a very characteristic appearance with abundant agranular cytoplasm and a large, often kidney-shaped, nucleus. The cytoplasm often shows several vacuoles.

131. This is a burr cell or echinocyte. This is one of the red-cell abnormalities characterised by the presence of spicules on the red-cell surface (the other is the acanthocyte). Burr cells have more spicules which are shorter and broader in comparison to the acanthocyte. The red cell may also be irregularly contracted. These cells are most commonly seen in renal failure but may be found in a wide variety of other conditions including pyruvate kinase deficiency and lipid abnormalities. Burr cells should be distinguished from crenated red cells which are an artefact of storage and are characterised by many small fine projections on an essentially normally shaped red cell.

132. This is a basophil. These cells are the least common of the white cells in the peripheral blood and are characterised by deeply basophilic coarse granules. Basophils are increased in chronic granulocytic leukaemia, although in this situation their granulation is often defective and the cytoplasm may contain only a few granules revealing a kidney-shaped nucleus.

133. This is a late normoblast characterised by well haemoglobinised cytoplasm and a small pyknotic nucleus. This is the last stage of red-cell development in the marrow. Occasionally these cells are seen in the peripheral blood, e.g. normally in neonates and fetuses, but may also be a sign of marked erythroid-cell stimulation, e.g. in severe hypoxia or bleeding or when a tumour exists in the marrow.

134. Intermediate normoblast. In this cell the nucleus still retains some open chromatin and the cytoplasm, although well haemoglobinised, retains a basophilic tinge. Active haemoglobin production still occurs at this stage.

135. This is an erythroblast. It is characterised by a large nucleus with open chromatin and basophilic cytoplasm and few granules. There may be an easily identified Golgi zone. This is an early stage of erythroid development. Haemoglobin production has probably not started at this point. The basophilic nature of the cytoplasm is due to the large amounts of RNA required for haemoglobin production. Ferritin granules can be seen on electron microscopy which also reveals many mitochondria.

136. This is a metamyelocyte. This is the last stage of neutrophil production in the marrow. The tertiary granules are now well formed. The nucleus, which has no nucleoli, has a distinct horseshoe shape although segmentation has not yet started, which is the next stage in the development of these cells. In B12 and folate deficiency, giant forms of metamyelocytes, which are end cells and incapable of further development, are seen and may persist for up to seven days following the correction of B12 and folate deficiency.

137. This is a myelocyte. After this stage of neutrophil development there is no further cell division. The nucleus which is eccentric starts to become kidney shaped. Secondary granules are well formed although some primary granules may be seen scattered throughout the cytoplasm. Secondary granules of neutrophil series contain lactoferrin and B12 binding proteins as well as lysozyme, which is also seen in primary granules. There is some dispute as to whether secondary and tertiary granules are distinct entities.

138. This is a promyelocyte. In normal promyelocytes the nucleus is eccentric. The chromatin pattern is still open and the nucleoli are seen. These cells are capable of division. Primary granulation is very prominent as is the Golgi zone. Primary granules of neutrophil series, most readily seen in the promyeloctye, contain mainly lysozyme, other enzymes such as acid phosphatase and myeloperoxidase. These play a role in bacterial killing which is one of the important functions of the neutrophil.

139. This is a megakaryocyte. These are very characteristic cells which are rarely mistaken. The cells are hyper-diploid and may have up to 32 nuclei. The cytoplasm in mature forms is granular and may even be seen to be budding platelets, although this is probably an *in vitro* artefact caused by the preparation of the marrow films.

140. This is a marrow macrophage which, in this case, shows some haemosiderin. These are relatively common cells which appear to have a role in scavenging cell debris and, in particular, iron from cells. Marrow macrophages probably also play a role in transferring iron to developing normoblasts.

Index

Numbers refer to the number shared by the illustration, question and answer.